BUSY BODY

First published in 2006 by Fusion Press,
a division of Satin Publications Ltd
101 Southwark Street
London SE1 0JF
UK
info@visionpaperbacks.co.uk
www.visionpaperbacks.co.uk
Publisher: Sheena Dewan

Author's note:
In some cases, names and identifying characteristics have been
changed to protect the privacy of the individuals involved.

A catalogue record for this book is available from the British Library.

ISBN: 1-904132-94-4

2 4 6 8 10 9 7 5 3 1

Cover and text design by ok?design
Printed and bound in the UK by Mackays of Chatham Ltd,
Chatham, Kent

This book is dedicated with love to
Marianne Bloss, Dennis Bloss, Susanna Bloss
and to M de B — my soul mate.
And to all the millions of people
who have Tourette's syndrome.
God knows we're slightly different,
but who said different is bad?

A wise man should consider that health is the greatest of human blessings, and learn how by his own thought to derive benefit from his illnesses.

Hippocrates (460–377 BCE)

CONTENTS

	Acknowledgements	xi
	Prologue	1
CHAPTER 1:	Welcome	7
CHAPTER 2:	Tic, Tic, Tic . . .	11
CHAPTER 3:	I *Have* to	17
CHAPTER 4:	The Power of Touch	23
CHAPTER 5:	Ants in his Pants	33
CHAPTER 6:	Woof, Woof	41
CHAPTER 7:	Institutional Bullying	51
CHAPTER 8:	Numbers, Things, Details	63
CHAPTER 9:	Touch Heaven	71
CHAPTER 10:	Detective Work	81
CHAPTER 11:	A Brain in Conflict	91

CHAPTER 12: **One Last Word** 99

CHAPTER 13: **Transition** 105

CHAPTER 14: *I'll* **Show You Obsessions** 121

CHAPTER 15: **Pandemonium** 129

CHAPTER 16: **A Revelation** 143

CHAPTER 17: **A Peculiar Syndrome** 149

CHAPTER 18: **The Temple** 155

CHAPTER 19: **All at Sea** 167

CHAPTER 20: **So Close to Success** 177

CHAPTER 21: **Burning Bridges** 187

CHAPTER 22: **Death at the Door** 195

CHAPTER 23: **Radioactive Tourette's** 203

CHAPTER 24: **Drill Sergeant** 213

CHAPTER 25: **Full Circle** 223

Epilogue 235

About the Author 241

ACKNOWLEDGEMENTS

Although the actual act of penning *Busy Body* was an entirely solitary process – one in which I was both researcher *and* research material – the result of my efforts would not have been possible had it not been for the help of a number of people.

My agent, Peter Buckman, had faith in the book from its earliest stage and wholeheartedly encouraged me in its completion. He provides an unending supply of astute comments and advice, and possesses the uncanny gift of always being right. I'm in very safe hands.

Working with the spirited team at Fusion Press was a joy, and I'd like to express my appreciation to the whole crew – with special thanks going to Sheena Dewan, my publisher, for her belief in the book and also for letting me grab her elbows with all ten fingers; commissioning editor Charlotte Cole, for her tremendous enthusiasm; Louise Coe for meticulously editing and patiently helping me clarify my own thoughts in order to pull the book into shape; Sam Evans for being so thorough with publicity; and Paul Swallow and Katie Davison for all their hard work on the sales front.

The following also deserve to be mentioned: Alan Morrison for listening patiently as I incessantly prattled on about the past; Carolyn Kotok, for her solid-as-a-rock friendship; Vitor (the dentist) Salgueiro, for his cosy calm, not to mention an attempt at providing me with Tourette-proof teeth; Fiona York for being so understanding and lovely in every sense; George Yiannorides for laughing *with* me and *at* me; Nuno Moura for his loyalty and colourful debate on stoicism and the like.

Thank you all.

PROLOGUE

The gate clicked shut behind me and I started counting. My pace was steady, and anyone who might have been watching me on that particular Wednesday morning would have seen just another teenager on his way to school, weaving through the bustling North London streets, neither hurrying nor dawdling. I had made the same journey hundreds of times and knew that it took between 2,200 and 2,283 steps, no more and no less – although, since my route never varied, I had never quite worked out why there was such a difference between the two figures.

The day had started out like all others. I'd woken to my clock radio blaring out some breakfast programme at 7.45 am and reluctantly heaved myself out of bed. A quick 'Hello' to my mother, as I went down four staircases and forty-four stairs, and I was in the kitchen boiling a kettle for some tea and ignoring, as always, the packet of cereal that had been put out for me the previous night. My stomach was already starting to twinge with nerves; there was just no way I was going to attempt to force food down my throat.

As I stood in the kitchen I smashed my upper teeth hard against my lower, time and time again with a precise motor rhythm, and when that pattern seemed to be nicely established I was made to add a hard and violent nodding of my head to the mix, which seamlessly joined and became one with the jaw smashing.

Tea in hand, I went back upstairs to take a quick shower, during which I inevitably caught sight of myself in the mirror and my heart sank as I realised that there had been no miraculous overnight improvement in my looks and that I was still pretty gross. Peering into the mirror, I saw my eyes twitching and watched with mild fascination as the twitch evolved, as usual, into a hard blinking, which made me screw my eyes up as tightly as possible. I saw some head nodding and watched my face contort painfully as I smashed my jaws together. I shook my head violently from side to side and then saw just how ridiculous I looked when I nodded at myself. I heard a little voice in my head say, 'You ugly freak!' and my near continuous nodding almost turned into a demented affirmation as I said back to myself, 'Yes, you really are.'

As I dressed, and nodded and shook my head and blinked and smashed my teeth together, I was aware of an almost imperceptible crescendo in the noises that had begun so softly. At a rate of once every seven seconds or so, I made a short and intense sort of high-pitched 'ooh' sound, which by the time I was half dressed had turned into a 'pah'. I mentally logged that my shirt had seven buttons as I fastened them and, just before I threw on a sweater, I was forced to punch myself hard in the stomach five times.

My shoes were always a nightmare. Sitting on my bed, I tied and untied my laces ten times in succession and, when something in my brain told me that they were in fact well and truly tied, I had to feel my way around the shape of the tip of each shoe, with my fingers all bunched up together and applying equal force as they journeyed around the leather.

I gave my hair a bit of a ruffle, took another quick look in the mirror, nodded and blinked a few times back at myself and I was ready.

I went down the stairs again, two at a time this time and therefore only twenty-two stairs, dashed to the front door, picked up my school bag and flung it over my shoulder, called out a quick goodbye and I was on the street.

Walking along, my brain clicked on to automatic and began clocking my steps, allowing me the chance to start my mental prayer routine. It wasn't that I was religious in any organised sense of the word; it was more a prayer borne from a deeply held belief that if I implored hard enough to a higher authority – *any* higher authority – then someone or something somewhere might eventually hear me. My imploring was so intense and my concentration so great that I was almost unaware of any nodding, shaking, blinking or noises that I might have been forced to execute.

As I neared the school gates, and the reality of what I was about to have to go through yet again loomed large, my praying became more fervent. 'Please don't let them hurt me, please make my nerves stop, please don't let me cry, please don't let them notice me today, please, please, please . . .' The butterflies in my stomach seemed to be somersaulting, and I fought a wave of nausea as I tried to get a grip and order myself, as I did each day, to just be normal.

I felt a hard blow to my right arm, a 'dead arm' they called it, and the pain seared through me, and then someone spat at me and I felt the saliva run down my forehead. Another school day had begun.

The day dragged on like all others. Drab lessons given by fittingly drab teachers all took place in the constant company of aggressive teenagers, who, to my mind, acted as if they had somehow got stuck near the bottom rung of Darwin's evolutionary scale. I sat alone in most lessons and when the bell went for morning break, I dashed to a toilet on the third floor, one that I hoped would be deserted, and locked myself in a cubicle and allowed myself to shake and nod and flex and blink, all the things that I'd had to try so hard to make less obvious in class. At lunchtime I managed to find an empty corner on one of the back stairways, and there I stood like a sentry, listening and watching for any sign that someone may be approaching, always ready to retreat further to some other secluded spot that I had already deemed safe.

The highlight of the day, for everyone else at least, was a weekly occurrence directly after lunch, before the last lesson of the day. It was called 'form period' and was a time when, as a form, we were supposed to sit quietly with our form teacher and chat, either to her or among ourselves. The role of a form teacher was to deal with the pastoral care side of things, to converse with us, make sure everything was going well, or to help solve things if they were not. However, my particular teacher rarely had any interpersonal exchange with any of those in her care; she used to sit doing her own thing during form periods while the rest of the class did theirs.

I remember being jostled in line before form period that day. Someone thumped me and someone else had mimicked my facial tics and called me a fucking animal, much to the amusement of everyone else who still laughed at a term that had been applied to me thousands of times before.

During form period I sat alone. The desks were arranged in a horseshoe around the teacher and my place was right on the end, with an empty space next to me because no one wanted to be near me. Our teacher took the register and then gave her usual command of, 'Chat quietly among yourselves,' and form period began.

As always, I sat and concentrated on my body. I willed it to stay calm and still, tried with all my might to stifle my tics and violent head-shaking and nodding and kept a mental 'no, no, no' going, anything to stop attention being drawn to me. The other kids were joking about and chatting to each other, and our teacher was busying herself with marking exercise books.

Then it happened.

I felt a welling up of energy from somewhere deep inside my body and I made a huge and loud 'ooh' sound – a yelp. It was a noise that was a constant in my life, one that I absolutely had to make, and one over which I had no control whatever. I just couldn't help it. I could fight some of my inevitable noises some of the time, or at least I could take the edge off their violence, but this was one of my biggies, and as soon as I felt that familiar and relentlessly rising force of energy I knew exactly what was about to happen. I could do nothing to stop its release.

My form teacher looked at me and sarcastically asked if I had something that I wanted to say. The room went quiet and all eyes were on me. I couldn't answer. I had no words. The teacher told me to stand up and I did. She asked me again whether I had something to say and I still remained silent. There were giggles around the room and then that wonderfully hushed sense of anticipation that occurs when everyone just knows that something is about to happen. My teacher told me to remain standing until I had an answer to her question. I was ticcing furiously now. I was quivering. Up and down went my head, my eyes blinked harder than they ever had before, and I made little vocal noises.

Suddenly, a boy raised his hand to ask the teacher a question. The teacher looked at him and nodded for him to go ahead. 'What I'd like to know,' he said, 'is why he barks like a dog.' Laughter. Another question, 'Can we ask him to blink for us?' *More.* 'He thinks he's an animal.' *More.* 'He *is* an animal.' *More.* 'Hey, Freaky, bark for us.' *More.* 'He's so blind and ugly, look how he nods.' *More.* 'Look at Noddy, look at Noddy.' *More.* 'Hey, freaky boy.' *More.* 'He's soooooooooo nervous.' *More.* 'Nod for us Noddy, nod for us.' *More.* 'Look how he's batting his eyelids, he thinks he's pretty.' *More.* 'Pretty doggy, pretty doggy.' *More.* 'Blinkerrrrrrrrr.' *More.* 'Why does he have to be in our class?' *More.* 'He should be at a school for retards.' *More. And more. And more. And more. And more . . .*

Everyone was screaming with laughter. It was deafening. They were stamping their feet. They were standing and pointing menacingly. Their voices spiralled around me like a demented whirlwind, their warped and mocking faces kept shooting into my vision. I saw spit as it was lobbed across the room at me and I felt the wetness as it landed.

I looked at the teacher for help, but she too was laughing. In fact, she was in stitches and almost convulsing.

I remained standing.

As I stood there, the tears poured down my cheeks.

Chapter 1

Welcome

As I swing the doors to my world wide open, I hope that you'll come in and take a good look at all the peculiar layers of strange and exhausting clutter that make up my existence. You see, I'm a blinking, nodding, yelping, snorting, raspberry-blowing, tooth-grinding, jaw-smashing, nail-biting, buttock-clenching, hyperventilating, head-shaking, squinting, grimacing, pouting, counting, spitting, touching, knee-bending, calf-flexing, stomach-contracting, laughing and obsessing sort of character. That's the fundamental 'me' in my dealing with the bombardment of strident sounds, blinding sights, potent smells, accusing looks, tempting-to-touch surfaces and booming voices that mercilessly rain on me from your world, resulting in frustration, suppression, anguish, pain, insult, aching, side-splitting-hysteria, nervousness, fatigue and ultimately a desperate, yet smotheringly chaotic, sense of isolation.

Welcome to the dizzy world of Tourette's syndrome!

Tourette's syndrome? Oh yeah, that weird thing that makes me swear all the time at everything, everyone and anyone.

That quirky illness that gives me the excuse to pluck almost my whole vocabulary from the mountainous piles of invective available to us all, if only we dare use them. That wonderful syndrome that allows me to call a policeman a four-eyed, worthless, mother-fucking bastard, *and* get away with it.

Wrong!

I do not swear and gush expletives because I have Tourette's syndrome. In fact I probably swear no more and no less than you do. Not all people who have Tourette's syndrome swear, and swearing *does not* solely characterise this unusual syndrome. Statistically, only a small number of people with Tourette's display the signs of this extremely bizarre and inconvenient 'strain' of it, and I'm sure none of us can imagine how distressing it must be to have literally no control over the severity and frequency of expletives that seem to flow effortlessly from the tongue. It is a little sad, though, that the sole portrayal of people with Tourette's consists of films, plays, books, articles and popular characterisation of sad, foul-mouthed and confused little creatures with no control over what they say. It really paints the wrong picture. Incidentally, the technical name for this occasional symptom of Tourette's is 'coprolalia', but I fondly refer to it as PMT, or Potty Mouth Tourette's.

Since PMT doesn't (thankfully) feature big time in my world, I'm not going to harp on about it, in case I end up fully developing it, as it's not an uncommon phenomenon among Tourette people to 'adopt' things that are suggested to them, or to end up aping the behaviour of others.

Tourette's syndrome seems to be almost fashionable these days, or at least the name is. Although I personally like to call sufferers Tourettists, which, to me, sounds almost as innocuous as motorist, philanthropist or even florist, the word Tourette's pops up all the time, on the radio, on television and in the papers. Whereas if I'd told anyone ten years ago that I was a Tourette's sufferer I could have expected a blank stare in return, the name now seems to actually register with some people. Many react as if I'd said that I had two heads, while others almost visibly 'duck' to avoid the expected onslaught of verbal abuse. What *is* strange is that Tourette's seems to have become almost trendy. That's not to suggest anyone actually wants to have it. It's kinkier than that. Some people seem to get off on the idea of knowing a Tourettist. For example, I turned up at a dinner party recently and the host, loudly and proudly and with a wonderfully hammed-up French accent, announced that I had 'La Tourette's'. A multitude of 'ooh's and 'aah's reverberated around the room and everyone converged on me as though I was royalty. By the end of the night various people had my phone number in order to invite me to their homes, where they, no doubt, thought they would metaphorically poke, prod and examine me under that wonderful human microscope called fascination. I was a specimen. I was an oddity. I was suddenly a party accessory.

So why am I writing this? Why am I attempting to show you how life is as a Tourettist? Well, I could go down Politically-Correct Avenue now and say that I want people to see beyond the Tourette's, to understand and see me and all other Tourettists as valid and worthy human beings. True as all that may be, I'm afraid that the PC approach really doesn't do it for me and I'm certainly not looking for sympathy either.

What I would like to do is to describe in no-nonsense, non-medical, non-bleeding-heart, non-politically correct and non-mumbo-jumbo language *exactly* what it is like to have Tourette's. I want you to get to know me as a Tourettist.

CHAPTER 2

TIC, TIC, TIC...

I'm sure you've sat on a bus, in a restaurant or on the train immersed in your own thoughts, happily minding your own business, when suddenly something somewhere catches your eye. To be more precise, *someone* catches your eye. You're not quite sure why, but you focus on that someone and to your mild fascination they tic right there before your very eyes. Maybe it was a quick wink of the eye, something that might have been construed as a cheeky come-on if it happened just the once, but every five seconds or so . . . no way. Maybe it was a series of exaggerated frowns, or a speedy but continuous rabbit-like crinkling of the nose. A few ups and downs from the eyebrows, or even just the one eyebrow? Odd little nods of the head? Or maybe it was a straining of the eyes, first to the left, then painfully all the way back to the right, or – cleverest of all – completely crossed or even diagonally opposite.

It's quite amazing that a seemingly harmless little tic can precipitate all manner of emotions in others. If you were to describe that stranger who ticced for you then you might say something along the lines of, 'I saw this guy earlier with the most *horrendous* tic,' or, 'That woman pulled such *hilarious* faces,' or even, 'Jeez, it's amazing the number of loons they let out these days.' But, and this is a big but, if you're talking about someone you actually know who has a tic, then the emotional pull of your vocabulary changes entirely. You'll either paint a colourful picture by saying something like, 'My friend so-and-so has all *manner* of weird and wonderful eccentric tics,' or you'll go down the bleeding-heart path and say, 'Such-and-such suffers *terribly* from her nerves. God, she has dreadful nervous tics.' Well, true, someone may appear somewhat nervous or eccentric because of their particular tic, but I'm certain it takes more than a harmless little tic to make a fully-fledged nervous wreck or eccentric. I say, take the nervous out of the tic. So what if someone has a tic or three? Tics are harmless. For the vast majority of people a tic doesn't ruin their lives or consume them during every waking moment. Now the tics of a seasoned Touretterist are a completely different ball game. A full-blown Touretterist tics *all the time* he or she is awake. There is no respite, no brief let-up and absolutely no controlling them. Just as you breathe and blink without a thought, so the Touretterist tics.

Here's a little exercise:

Keeping your eyes wide open, do not allow yourself to blink. Not even a little blink, not even the once. Gets uncomfortable, doesn't it? You feel something, an energy almost, surging up from deep within you, although you are not quite sure where this energy comes from or what exactly it is. It tempts you at first, then it absolutely compels you to blink. No matter how strong you are, how controlled, how mind-over-matter detached, you just know that you are going to have give in to the demands of your own body, which will be silently screaming orders at you, and blink. There is nothing you can do about it. Please remember that feeling, that suspense, that welling up of compelling energy, that merciless order from deep within to blink whether you want to or not. That is how a Tourettist feels if he or she tries to stifle a tic.

Oh, but if only it was just the one tic.

I worked out that I tic, somewhere in my body, about forty times a minute. That's 2,400 tics an hour, so if I'm awake for the usual sort of sixteen-hour day, then I tic somewhere in the region of 38,400 times a day. Now that's one hell of a load of ticcing and, like you if you try not to blink, there is nothing I can do the stop the damn things.

I tried to think of the most effective way to describe my tics and movements as they are right now. My first thought was creating a kind of a 'tic diary', but on reflection I would have gone completely and utterly mad trying to document even a day's worth. Half a day then? After all, you really have no idea what a professional ticster like me is all about. How about an hour, or even just fifteen minutes? No! Far too lengthy and complicated. So I've settled on just one measly little minute. Pen in hand and one eye on the second hand of my clock, I'll try and describe what's going on as I try and write, here and now. Here goes:

Buttocks clench four times in succession, then the left one once, then the right one twice – left forearm flexes, then the right, then both together four times – calves at it now, flex and let go, flex and let go – a few rapid, but hard blinks of the eyes – five trademark shakes of the head – buttocks again – now the tummy, pull it all the way in as hard as possible, then all the way out, straining with all my might – back teeth in, upper and lower jaws smashed together hard – stomach again – calves – big toe on each foot up and down – a shake of the head – two hard blinks – eyes crossed, just the once, thankfully – balls of both feet pressed hard into the floor, seven times in rapid succession for some strange reason and accompanied by a head-shake and a smashing of teeth . . . Ah, but only thirty seconds have passed . . . on . . . a dash of a calf flex, another rapid shake of the head, which really hurt, two forearm shakes, five teeth smashes, four buttock clenches – up and down, up and down, up and down, up and down – two tight pursings of the lips, a hint of a head-shake, tummy in and out twice and big toe of right foot up and down three times and . . . the minute's up.

You think I'm kidding around, don't you? I wish I could say that I was. In fact, if anything, I probably left a few tics out of that tiny little minute, not being able to recognise and register one tic before another had taken over. And remember, I'm only talking about the tics – I deliberately left out all of the other Touretty things that were going on.

'Nonsense,' you might well say. 'If he really tics like that he wouldn't be able to function normally.' Not so. I function just fine, thanks. In my world, that is. It's all so normal for me. However, if I had a magic wand and could suddenly make you tic as I do, then I'm pretty sure you'd probably keel over with exhaustion in the first hour. So am I saying I'm some kind of superman and stronger than all of you? No, I'm not. Remember the blinking exercise? Well, you blink naturally (as do I), but I also tic just as naturally. My tics are as compulsory to me as blinking or breathing is to you. But here's the problem – my problem. Whereas blinking or breathing causes no pain, no exhaustion, no embarrassment and no discomfort, the tics, while being no less avoidable for me, are another matter.

The constant activity is shatteringly exhausting. My body inflicts pain on itself by forcing me to do things time and time again, never showing the slightest hint of mercy. Just have a go at shaking *your* head with all your might and jerking your neck at the same time and rolling your eyes hard back in their sockets, and try telling me that it doesn't hurt. The problem is that I cannot NOT tic and the harder I try not to, the more urgent the need to tic becomes.

Apart from the fact that, since I have no control over these tics, they become a huge embarrassment and people often gawp at me and treat me like I'm the village idiot – something I'm kind of used to now – there's one thing about them that drives me to despair. I cannot escape from myself, from the me of constant activity, movement, clenching, grinding, flexing, shaking, pulling and pushing. One thing I cannot do is relax. Please don't tell me to sit still, because I simply can't. It's impossible for me to vegetate on the sofa and read a book or watch television in peace. I just can't take time off from myself, however desperately I might want to.

Consciously trying to relax seems to make me less inhibited and therefore the tics gang up on me and play havoc with me when my defences are down. Engaging in some tiring activity certainly tires my body, but unfortunately does nothing to calm the tics. They seem to love taking advantage of me when I have little energy to fight them back. There is unfortunately no solution – I cannot win, cannot escape and cannot conquer the exhausting and exhaustive movements of my own body.

And so it goes.

So when did I start all this ticcing? How did it all begin? Funnily enough, I remember it like it was yesterday. I was all of seven years old, walking from the lounge to the kitchen via the hallway, when it happened. No glamorous setting for *my* first tic, no wonderfully traumatic or harrowing event to act as a catalyst, nothing and no one for me to blame, just a simple stroll though an average hallway. I stopped, screwed up my eyes as tightly as possible whilst rolling my eyeballs painfully in their sockets and simultaneously shaking my head from left to right twice in rapid succession. There it was. The first tic. After thirty years I'm still at it and not a day has gone by when I haven't done it.

Now, painful and embarrassing as that head-shaking tic became, the tic story didn't end there. Far from it. In fact, it was the tic from which all of my tics were born. It was just a beginning.

CHAPTER 3

I *HAVE* TO

So, at seven years old, I found myself shaking my head vigorously and continuously. It hurt, but I couldn't help myself. My parents, quite naturally, became alarmed. It was all so sudden. 'What are you doing?', 'What *is* it?', 'Is something wrong?', 'Don't do that, darling!', 'STOP IT!' I heard these words time and time again, but could give no response, except to favour everyone with another violent head-shake.

I overheard my parents talking about it, my mother crying. Questions, questions, questions. 'Is it nerves?', 'Could it be food additives?', 'Is it something we're doing?', 'Is it brain damage?', 'Is he OK at school?' Questions that stayed unanswered. More tears. More anxiety. More questions.

I was duly taken to our family doctor. I vividly recall him asking me to 'perform' for him, but I couldn't. I clammed up. My enemy, my shaking head, went suddenly inert. The doctor looked dubious. I wanted to scream at him as he peered at me over his glasses as though I was an unattractive little specimen in a jar. 'Help me,' I wanted to say. 'Please make it go away.' But I was too scared. I was seven.

The general consensus seemed to be that whatever it was that I was doing, I would 'grow out of it'. God, was that an expression I would have to get used to hearing. Actually, for a while things did seem to stabilise. That's not to say the head-shaking stopped, it just didn't seem to be getting more aggressive. But then, almost out of the blue, I developed more 'things'. Crossing my eyes, jerking my neck round and round, nodding my head. Suddenly, these became part of me too. What I now know was Tourette's syndrome was taking hold and whetting its greedy, perverse, chemical, neuro-transmittery appetite, and, while my family seemed to think – or at least hope – I would 'grow out of it', I instinctively knew that things were not going to be that simple.

I started doing new and stranger things – like jumping up and making sure that in mid-air both of my feet would slap hard against my buttocks at exactly the same time. This would occur countless times each day. Then I had to do this jump-kick thing a certain number of times in succession – say fifty – and if my feet happened not to strike my buttocks simultaneously then I would have to start the count again from scratch. It was exhausting. I was confused. I was embarrassed. I was scared and I had no way of explaining to my startled family why I was behaving in such a way. All I could say was, 'I *have* to.'

My class teacher at school became concerned and spoke to my parents about my 'odd' behaviour. My friends wondered what the hell I was doing, and those who were not my friends began to mock and imitate me. My little world was turning upside-down and I had no idea why. All I knew was that it wasn't my fault.

My parents gave me all the love and understanding that they could, but what was there to pinpoint or to understand? No one had the faintest hint of an idea as to what was going on with me. In any case, my parents had other problems. My brother, Jeremy – ten years older than me and a phenomenally gifted pianist – had become a heroin addict. He was not living with us then, and my poor parents lived in fear for him. As they waited for news of Jeremy, they watched me jumping, kicking, blinking and head-shaking, and were helpless in both situations.

A referral in 1976 to a hospital paediatric neurology specialist finally bore fruit. 'It's nerves,' the learned doctor rather predictably pronounced. 'They are nervous tics. We'll start him on Valium. He'll grow out of it.' I was eight years old, sentenced to Valium and toddled off, pills in hand, in the hope of miraculous results. In truth though, I never took the Valium, although I led everyone to believe I was giving it a go. The problem was I just couldn't swallow the pills: they wouldn't go down. I'd had no experience of downing pills and I simply didn't know how to do it effectively; the harder I tried to swallow, the more bitter the taste of the dissolving pill became and I'd end up gagging. Now if I'd been given Valium in a pleasant tasting elixir I might have even enjoyed taking it, but the sour pills were all that was offered. I might have been just eight, but I knew I wasn't going to persevere with something so unpleasant. So each day when it was time to take my pill, glass of water in hand, I'd throw it behind a particularly large chest freezer in our kitchen when no one was looking and then triumphantly produce the empty glass and give an 'I've taken it' look of satisfaction. Years later when the freezer had to be moved for some reason, hundreds of little white pills were discovered piled up behind it. I gave everyone my best innocent look and disappeared to my room as fast as I could.

My little world became busier by the day. Head-shaking was soon complemented by vicious head-nodding – a sharp downward nod with my chin hitting my thorax, hard. Punching myself in the stomach became satisfying – right hand, thumb knuckle bent to a point, hard. I felt myself nodding, punching and the rest, and tried to work out why. But I always drew the same conclusion: because I had to. It was all so necessary. It all seemed so perfectly right in a blatantly wrong kind of way.

My parents, who still believed that I was taking the Valium, tried very hard to get to the root of the problem, to solve it. It wasn't their fault they failed. My mother delicately counselled me, probing as much as you can into an eight-year-old mind, to see if there was anything disturbing me. Nothing was, except the tics. I was a lively, confident, well-adjusted, bright and happy child, sensitive and doing well at school. My father had the ingenious idea of timing me and seeing how long I could go without a tic, rewarding me with a penny for each minute that went by without incident. So I concentrated like crazy whilst picturing a bursting piggy bank. And, funnily enough, I did manage to go for many minutes without much tic activity. 'Ah,' you're all saying, 'so he *could* control it.' Well yes, and no. I didn't know then how or why I could stifle the tics, but recent research has shown that Tourettists can stifle tics, or rather it's not the Tourettist who does the stifling, but the brain itself. Apparently, when a Tourettist focuses 110 per cent on something or is distracted to the point of absolute concentration, the brain releases a chemical that seems to stop, or certainly decrease, the severity of the tics. Why the brain does this no one can satisfactorily say, but it does. Well, sometimes it does. Still, none of my family had any idea about that then. We never knew that such a thing as Tourette's syndrome existed. I was just a boy with 'bad nerves'.

Chapter 4

The Power of Touch

Touch is, for some Tourettists, perhaps the most potent, all-consuming and heightened sense they have. After all, fingers really are quite remarkable little things and the great thing about them is that they sit at the ready all day, every day, poised to leap into action for you. They enable you to grab, scratch, fumble, hold a pen, turn on the tap, pick your nose, drive your car, feel the quality of material, determine whether something is hard or soft or dry or lumpy and on and on and on. I'll bet you never even give these incredible little wonders so much as a thought. You never think, 'Right, fingers at the ready, I'm about to pick up my car keys,' or, 'Gosh, I've got an itchy leg, now I'll just extend my index finger so I can use it for a jolly good scratch.' In fact, most people ignore their fingers almost entirely and rarely give them any particular attention.

But it's very different where my fingers are concerned. It's all to do with my awareness of my fingers – the digits themselves and what they do best: touch. You see, I touch things much more than you do. Believe me, I do. Yes, of course you touch things all day long, as we all do. Fingers make contact with something or someone hundreds and hundreds of times a day. You aren't even aware what they are going to touch, or how many times they are going to touch. In fact, most of the time you are not really registering exactly what it is you are touching. If I were to ask you what things you've touched today, I'd be willing to bet that you couldn't give anything like a precise answer. But if you asked me, *I* could.

Just as I cannot stifle a tic, nor can I stifle the need to touch particular things. There's no reasoning to it. But it's more than just a little compulsion and much more than a mere touchy-feely quirk. It's an absolute necessity. It is as vital to my well-being to have to touch various things as blinking is to yours. Believe me, it's not that I actually *want* to touch certain things in order to have a bloody good feel. I *have* to.

So what are these wonderful things that I have to touch? Well, before I answer that I'd better explain exactly what touch means for me, because it's almost certainly different to your perception of it. I don't touch something for just a fraction of a second, without thought or meaning. Nor do I gracefully let my fingers waft in an affected manner over the surface of something. My touch isn't delicate or subtle. When I talk about touching something, I mean that I place all ten fingers on whatever it is that has caught my eye and either press it really hard if it's a tough item, or grab it with all ten fingers and have a wonderfully satisfying squeeze if it's in any way flexible. Sounds simple, doesn't it? Well, I'm afraid, like the best things in life, it isn't.

Some things are actually rather difficult to touch or grab effectively – a lift button, the head of a screw, the 'R' key on a computer keyboard, a garden pea, the rim of a delicate crystal glass, the picture rail seven feet above ground in my lounge, the wobbly surface of a freshly baked soufflé. Some things are painful to touch – the hot electric ring on the cooker, the shell of a newly boiled egg, a light bulb when it is switched on, a wonderfully tempting shard of china from a dropped plate, the edge of the blade of a really sharp knife. Other things, sadly, are almost impossible to touch – the windscreen wipers on my car when I'm actually driving, the cake behind the glass display in the baker's – or, most risky of all: your left ear lobe, the tip of your nose, your left eye or your bony knee, should I ever meet you.

Now, if and when I do touch something, it's got to be touched 'properly', or I have to do it again and again and again, until my fingers are satisfied and let me know that the touched item has indeed been well and truly touched. The recipe for a good touch goes something like this:

1) Spot the item to be touched – I have absolutely no idea how or why my brain makes the choice of the 'thing', I just obey.

2) Home in on the item or object in question. At this stage the nerve endings in the tips of my fingers feel as thought they are suddenly going to red alert. It's like holding a magnet towards something metallic; you know, that wibbly, wobbly, slightly hesitant and odd pull that occurs just before the metal thing leaps towards the magnet.

3) Make any necessary physical adjustments in order to get at whatever it is I have to touch. This can be quite a tricky operation, especially if the item in question

is located somewhere awkward, or is so tiny that I have to bunch my fingers up as tightly as possible to get at it.

4) Make contact. This is the hardest and potentially the most hazardous part. All ten fingers must 'land' on the object at exactly the same moment. No one finger can be tardy here. Assuming successful contact has been made, I then hold the position for a few seconds and press the pads of the tips of my fingers into the object – again with an equal amount of force, otherwise it's back to stage 3 again. Hard objects just get a good press, but slightly more flexible ones always deserve a bit of gentle manipulation, I think – a slight pull, push or bend.

5) Release the thing, pull away and get on with whatever it was that I was doing before my brain commanded me to go though the annoying procedure above. Until the next time . . .

It's not only *things* that whet my Touretty touchy appetite, though. People make wonderful targets, or rather various bits of various people do. Again, there seems to be no rhyme or reason for it. I don't favour people with particularly prominent features over those with regular ones, or blondes over brunettes, or even men over women. At least, I don't consciously. It all seems rather ad hoc to me, although I can't possibly believe that in the mushy layers of my brain anything remotely random is going on. *It* knows exactly what it's about, the problem is, *I* don't. I can meet reams of people who do nothing for me, who don't disturb any deep cell neurotransmitter brain activity that I'm aware of. And then, all of a sudden, completely out of the blue, I'm talking to some-one or happen to spot someone, and that's it. All hell breaks loose. I *have* to touch them, or at least try to. But brushing unnoticed against their clothing won't do at all. That just wouldn't satisfy my brain. Remember, I'm mega touch sensi-tive. So it's back to the fingers again. They start tingling and, as the old magnet sensation sets in, I know I'll have to try and touch the poor, oblivious individual with, yes, you've got it, all ten fingers – and hard! And what's more, by now my brain will have directed my eye to a particular part of the person's anatomy and will be trying to geographically manoeuvre my fingers towards it. This really isn't just an excuse for me to have a good old grope at someone. Thankfully, up to now, I haven't been 'instructed' to claw at anyone's private bits and I pray it stays that way. In any case, I suppose it's usually things that seem to stick out at me that I tend to go for, or rather things that my brain makes *seem* to stick out at me. I must confess, though, to having a particular penchant for greasy noses – they really get me going. Chins run at a close second, with ear lobes, jowls, napes of necks, eyelids, elbows and knees bringing up the rear.

The good thing is that I tend only to home in on just the one of those particular body parts on each 'selected' person. The not-so-good thing is that I rarely get to satisfy my com-pulsion, as I can hardly go up to someone and say, 'Sorry to bother you, but would you mind if I just grab your tempt-ingly greasy nose with all ten fingers?' You see the dilemma? And, again, like with the tics or object touching, if I don't go through with the compulsion – this order from my brain to touch – then I'm not a happy camper. Hard as it is, I know that I have to hold myself back and exercise restraint when dealing with other people. My brain then seems to punish me for not expending the touch energy and for exercising polite reserve. In retribution, I am generally made to tic more violently than usual. It's a no-win situation. I'm just thankful that there aren't too many of you out there who are chosen by my brain's little selection process for some touchy Touretty treatment.

Be that as it may, I have to admit that I do get the chance to vent my desire to touch people sometimes, as I have a few friends who don't mind having ten fingers coming at them on the odd occasion. My friend Alan is the most patient and for some reason my brain really likes making me touch him. Alan is my closest friend and we go back a long way from our years at college. With him, though, it's not just a compulsion to touch one thing – it's a case of multiple touches. He senses when I'm about to pounce and knows the routine off by heart. First I go for his left ear, then the right, then his nose, chin, forehead and finally his jowls. He's well trained, bless him, and he turns his head first to the right so I can do an ear lobe, then to the left, so I can do the other one, he lifts his head for the nose, higher for the chin, down for the forehead and square-on for the jowls. Not a word is usually spoken while I'm pressing and pulling various bits of him – it's done in almost meditative silence – and when we both know that it's over we continue nattering as though nothing has happened. It's like everything went on 'pause' for a few moments. Time stood still.

Not everyone is as accommodating as Alan, though, and I often find myself in difficult situations: either trying to talk my way out of why I suddenly touched someone, or trying to poise myself in a strategic position for a touch opportunity.

Take flying, for example. I know that during any flight I take my brain will tell me to touch the hair of a particular one of my unsuspecting fellow passengers. I try to hold back for as long as I can, but sooner or later I just have to get up out of my seat and go for the kill. I usually end up having to pretend to stumble as I teeter along down the aisle, lashing out with my fingers for a fleeting, but very satisfying, touch as I'm 'falling'. It generally works and thankfully my brain is usually kind to me and targets someone sitting on the aisle, although on occasion I have had to manipulate a fall across a row of seats to get to some inconsiderate person who opted for a window seat.

So, I touch things, objects, items and people. What else, then?

This is the not-so-nice bit and I'm almost ashamed to have to admit it, but I am often compelled to touch rather yucky things. Let me reiterate: I do not *want* to touch them – I *have* to. For example, a filthy, slimy washing-up cloth in someone's kitchen sink – yep, with all ten fingers. The bristles of the toothbrush of someone I barely know; the inside rim of a dirty cup in a coffee shop, one that I have no idea whose mouth has been on it; the lids of dustbins; fungi on a tree; a discarded tissue left on a tube train seat. All manner of really vile things, in fact. Thinking about it makes me feel quite sick, so I can only imagine the impression of me that you are getting now. Don't judge me badly, though. I have no choice in the matter. I'm a professional Tourettist. It's Tourette's syndrome that makes me touch these things, even when I have no desire to.

One last aspect of this Touretty touching thing is in fact for me the most irritating. I can deal with 'homing in' on targets to touch with all ten fingers, and I can handle the urge to touch real people and even the disappointment when I can't. I can even manage the yucky touching, as long as I have lots of antibacterial wipes in my pocket. What really gets me though, what really holds up my day is having to go back and touch things that I accidentally touch. Something registers somewhere in my brain, which in turn sends me back the order that the thing I accidentally touched, which I really didn't want to touch in the first place, wasn't touched properly. Did you get all that? Here are a few examples of this exasperating feature of my world:

Imagine that I go to my desk to get a pen – nothing complicated so far – but as I'm reaching for the pen my hand might accidentally brush ever so lightly against my computer monitor. My brain jolts to life and seems to take over my next actions: I have to put the pen down, position my hands, take aim at the monitor and then touch it with all ten fingers according to the rules. Then, and only then, can I try and pick up the pen again and go on my merry way. You see, it takes me maybe four times as long to get the pen as it should have.

Cluttered bathrooms are a particular nightmare for me. Again, don't ask me why, because only my brain knows the answer. If I visit someone and have to go off and use their bathroom for a call of nature I break out into a cold sweat if I walk in and see clutter – bottles, cosmetics, toiletries and the likes. God forbid that my hand accidentally brushes against something as I reach for the tap or a towel. I have to touch it properly of course, but because of the clutter and the close proximity of everything to everything else, I often find myself accidentally touching something else too, and from then on it's the snowball effect and I usually become so jumpy that everything topples over and I have to give every item a bloody good, ten-fingered, hard squeeze. Heaven only knows what people imagine I get up to in their bathrooms when I spend so long in them, or what they think when they go in to discover all of their cluttered things rearranged.

No one could possibly expect me to actually enjoy all this touching, and I don't, but it's not by any means the most distressing feature of having Tourette's. It's just irritating and time-consuming and, of course, like many other Touretty manifestations, it's totally off the wall.

What I've described are the touchy Tourettisms as they are right now – the 'matured' touch, if you like. I'm in touch with my touch. I sense it, I expect it and, as I live with it, it lives with me. Touch features big time in my world.

CHAPTER 5

ANTS IN HIS PANTS

Developing what I call Touchy Tourette's was a real handicap for a little eight-year-old. There I was, crossing my eyes, shaking my head, nodding, jumping, kicking and punching myself, trying to carry on the normal life of a child, trying to understand what was happening to me, aching from the physical effort of the tics, agonising over the pain I was so obviously causing my parents, and the touching starts. It was as though somewhere deep in my brain a button had been pressed. If I were in a position now to give you an exact medical, biological, chemical definition of what happened (which I'm not), no matter how technically I could dress it up, no matter how logical I could make it sound, it would always amount to the same thing: something was released, a connection was made, a circuit completed. The bottom line is that one day, out of the blue, I just started touching things. The bizarre thing is that even though the touching became an absolute necessity to me, *other* people didn't realise it was happening, because they only saw the ever-so-obvious tics. What they didn't see was me *feeling* my way around a new-found world of touch sensation. Even I didn't equate touching things with the tics. *They* were so explosive and consuming, whereas the touching started so very subtly. I didn't just go up to the first someone in sight and grab his or her nose with all ten fingers. Nor did I frantically grasp for things way out of my reach. I *explored* touch. I was compelled and forced to discover it and there was nothing violent or demonstrative about it. I just knew that I had to touch things. It was almost as if my fingers were trying things out, undergoing a little 'probationary' period, finding a way to learn to touch in the precise way that would satisfy my Touretty brain.

Little fleeting touches were a fascinating prelude to full-blown Touretty touching. A grasp at the hem of my mother's skirt as she passed by, gentle manipulation of our dog's silky ear, a quick prod at his wet nose, bathroom taps, my father's knee, all of my toys, carpet, tiles, wood, plastic . . . The result left me feeling somehow touch-satisfied, and nothing remotely disturbed me in my quest for touch opportunities. But my Touretty brain is greedy, you see. *It* wanted more and more. So many things to potentially touch and with my thus far rather limited repertoire, it got bored. It started to demand and crave specific things. One such example was the light switch in my bedroom. It was just about graspable, so I ended up holding on to it as though my life depended on it. Once my brain discovered that the switch not only went up and down, but, in doing so, made a satisfying click to boot, all hell broke loose. Up and down it went, again and again. It became a ritual, a necessity for me to grasp that godforsaken light switch with all ten fingers and click it on and off each time I entered my bedroom. No other light switch deserved my absolute homage or appealed to me on any level. In consequence, my days became even busier because of that switch, and at the peak of my 'light switch period' I had to click it up and down, on and off, one hundred times each time I went past it, never releasing my fingers even for a moment, never waning with the force of pressure behind each finger, never denying my brain its quirky little thrill.

With my light switch escapades, and the innumerable jumping, bum-slapping kick things adding to my already disturbing catalogue of violent tics, my parents sought more help.

I was taken back to the hospital specialist. It was becoming evident that I was not 'growing out of' my odd behaviour at all. In fact, it was quite clear that I was growing into more startling patterns, Valium or no Valium. The doctor, who had seemed quite nice on the previous visit, despite the bitter Valium, now seemed to me to be as disagreeable as the pills he so readily prescribed. He wasn't particularly nice to me or my mother this time. He gave me a quick examination and I did a little tic routine for him – I wasn't going to be caught out on that one again – and he said that I was attention-seeking and in need of some sort of psychological counselling. *Lovely*! I think that somewhere along the way my mother had told him about the problems with Jeremy and his heroin addiction and the doctor probably put two and two together and came up with five. I remember trying to overhear the hushed conversation with my mother and catching the odd word: '. . . heroin . . . drug addict . . . trauma . . . family . . . attention-seeking . . .' I wanted to tell him that indeed I did seek attention. I wanted *his* attention. I wanted all of his god-like medical knowledge to make it all just stop, to make me better. I recall opening my mouth to try and say something, but nothing came out.

The doctor proposed another means to a cure. He upped the Valium – he was barking up the wrong tree there – and told my mother *not* to give my tics, jumping or touching any attention. That would 'cure' me, he said.

As it was, my parents didn't follow the doctor's advice and 'ignore me'. Nor did they withdraw their attention or support. Love was poured on me and, in return, I tried my hardest to make the tics and touching less obvious at home. I knew all about Jeremy and his heroin problem, of course, and I saw how their worry for him was draining my parents. I myself saw Jeremy, doped out of his mind on one of his infrequent visits, fall right into his plate of dinner. I watched as he swore and cursed at my parents, threatening them, cajoling and intimidating. I saw the demise of the 'wunderkind' brother pianist as he turned into an abusive animal. I saw him lying unconscious in the gutter one day when I was walking home from the sweet shop with a friend, and I was too ashamed to say, 'Look, there's my brother.' There was no way to shield me from the pain, the ugliness and the anxiety. I saw it all. But none of it made me touch, tic, jerk, jump, kick and punch. None of it made me an attention-seeking little boy. None of it was the cause of my own personal agonies and shame. I'm sure that reading this, you could easily think that it's no wonder I had hideous tics and other problems. But the truth of it is that my traumas, and those which would so mould my future, were a direct result of having Tourette's syndrome. I was fighting an enemy from within, you see. An enemy that would prove to be undefeatable.

As my Tourette's became worse, as the tics increased in violence, and as my 'touching' became more profound, I gradually began to live in my own jumbled secret little world. It was a world of oddity. From being a gregarious and confident child I became shy and self-conscious.

My older sister, Susanna, seven years my senior, was strapping, self-assured, athletic and beautiful. She was the middle child and, on the face of it, the best adjusted of the three of us. Already a teenager, she was undoubtedly dealing with problems of her own relating to growing up. And, between one brother who was a junkie and another who was getting attention because of his nerves, I'm sure life can't have been that easy for her. There's nothing new about sibling rivalry as a concept and, although I'm sure Susanna never consciously intended to lash out at anyone, to me, that is exactly what seemed to happen. She turned against me, and any chance of closeness between us suddenly vanished as I became the subject of her scorn. On one occasion she even stood by and watched her sporty friends mock me for being so 'weak', and she herself called me 'Noddy'. Of course all siblings tease and mock each other at some point, but her teasing made me feel so utterly demoralised at a time when I was feeling bad enough about myself.

For safety I clung to my mother and she clung back, not only because she hated seeing my world turning upside-down, but also because she died a little each day as she saw Jeremy descend that helpless spiral of no return that seems to grip so many drug addicts.

An appointment for me with the Homeopathic Hospital left none of us any wiser. I was seen by a panel of men and remember being mildly fascinated because they all had beards, which became a bit of a temptation for me because I was dying to have a feel, a quick grasp at their whiskers, but I thought I might get a smack if I did, so I didn't. They were probably all vegetarian, anti-vivisectionists, Baroque-music listeners and 2CV drivers as well, but I didn't know enough of the world to be able to speculate so vividly then. In any case, they were so terribly dull that I nearly fell asleep as they nodded, hmm'd and ahh'd. Many scratchings of beards later they reached their verdict and we were given a wise – I'm sure – little lecture on diet and I was prescribed a homeopathic pill with a very funny name. The learned homeopaths put all my 'symptoms' down to 'bad nerves' (that old chestnut) and I even heard the hint of a sentence that ended with 'attention-seeking'. *Great!* 'Bad nerves' I could just about deal with, but 'attention-seeking'? No. I knew they were wrong, so *very* wrong. The only good thing that came out of that little visit were the pills themselves, which were sugar coated, rather like little sweeties, and a pleasure to swallow. Not that they made the remotest amount of difference to my as-yet unexplainable symptoms.

At home the anxiety over Jeremy escalated. He had gone from being just an addict into being a dealer as well. Susanna, in contrast, became more beautiful and sporty by the day. As well as being confident and gregarious, she was a wonderful swimmer and a champion in her age group, and, despite us having no friendly relationship, I was always oddly comforted by her presence in the house because there was always a wonderful smell of chlorine in the air from her damp hair, which made me feel rather tranquil and safe. Nonetheless, she happily embraced the notion that I was attention-seeking and unfortunately the sea between us widened.

Along with my tics, jumping, kicking and punching, I became even more Tourettily touchy. The light switch thing never really relented and I now had to touch almost everything in sight as well. Then a weird touch variation developed. On being put to bed each night, I started having to touch/ press/push the headboard of my bed. Nothing to write home about so far, but combine that touch/ press/push with having to shout out 'Goodnight!' simultaneously and things start getting out of hand. It was a nasty trick for my Touretty brain to play on me. A really evil one. I would touch my headboard, shout out 'Goodnight!' and get a polite 'Goodnight' or 'Goodnight, darling' in reply from my parents, who were now downstairs reading, watching television, chatting or doing whatever it is that parents do. Then I'd touch the headboard again and say 'Goodnight', wait for the response and then do it again, and again, and again . . . I could hear anger creeping into my parent's voices as they replied, and who could really blame them? Their gentle 'Goodnight, darling' eventually turned into an angry 'GOODNIGHT. GOODNIGHT. YES, FOR GOD'S SAKE GOOOOODNIIIIIGHT!' I remember being beside myself. I couldn't stop touching and goodnighting and I was scared of making my parents cross. Usually, after their final 'GOODNIGHT' I'd manage to hold back, but just for a little while. It kept welling up inside me, you see. I'd start again. I'd have to. A touch of the headboard and a whispered 'goodnight' with the whisper getting louder and louder on each repetition and of course my parents eventually heard me. A polite 'goodnight' from them started the whole cycle again, until thankfully, for everyone, I managed to fall asleep.

Ten years old, a seasoned ticster, a professional toucher, and still no letting up. Not even a hint of 'growing out of it'. Some days were less 'violent' than others. Even some weeks were better than others. But there was no pattern, no reason, no obvious or less obvious cause and no helping or hindering. I fell into my role as the boy with bad nerves who touched things a lot. I was the son with tics, the brother who craved attention and the school friend who, according to my chums at the time, had 'ants in his pants'. The problem was that in my own head I didn't really have any idea what I actually was. I knew that I was not normal. I knew that my parents worried about me. I knew that my sister didn't have much time for me. I kind of knew that my friends accepted me. I suppose I knew that I was becoming submerged in my own (Touretty) world, but I knew that I had to be. I didn't know anyone else who did the same odd things as me. Other people were all so calm and so wonderfully similar, so absolutely normal. *They* weren't doing the things that I did. I wondered why I was made so different and if somewhere along the road I had done something terribly wrong that I was now being punished for. At ten years old you don't think things through philosophically, so I just got on with life, tics and touching and all. I shook my head, jumped, kicked, counted, nodded, crossed my eyes and touched anything and everything that I could lay my hands on. But I was OK. OK in my own busy little world.

Chapter 6

Woof, Woof

Some of you will already be convinced that Tourettists do actually bark and see sense in my chapter title. Some of you may have even read accounts of barking Tourettists or have seen a recent television play that showed a sad male Tourettist conducting a rather unintelligible woofing conversation with a dog he happened to encounter. Well, let me put your minds at rest. We Tourettists do not think that we are dogs. We do not converse with dogs, we don't cock our legs and pee against trees and we don't bark when the doorbell rings. In fact, we have nothing at all in common with our canine friends. This chapter is all about verbal tics, vocal tics, sometimes known as phonic tics and often called 'vocalalia'.

You might wonder how a tic can possibly be vocal. Up until now, the tics I've been describing – the shaking, clenching, nodding, blinking etc – have all been bodily, or motor, tics. They go on and on like a motor and affect various parts of my body. Verbal, or phonic, tics are the noises that Tourettists make. The noises they *have* to make. They are very strange things indeed, these verbal tics. They encompass a plethora of sounds that may seem pretty random to the listener, but that are vital to, and specifically used by, Tourettists. Just like the bodily tics, the need for a Tourettist to tic verbally is no less compelling. They are ultimately uncontrollable and absolutely inevitable. As with the bodily motor tics, some Tourettists vocally tic more than others. I've met some Tourettists who have almost unnoticeable bodily tics, but appalling vocal ones, and vice versa. With me, the vocal tics have remained a constant, and seem to exist happily alongside their sister tics of my body. Oddly enough, since I began writing this book, my vocal tics have literally exploded. I just can't seem to shut up. It could be because I'm having to delve deep within myself to accurately depict my TS, or maybe my vocal tics are on some kind of perverse little ego-trip that I don't know of and are going berserk just to remind me to feature them big time in my writing. Tourette's syndrome is a very selfish condition, after all.

So what exactly are these noises that I have to make? How do they sound? Well, let's deal with the so-called 'barking' first, as it seems to be the one that is most often associated with Tourettists, even though, strictly speaking, it is nothing like a canine bark at all.

The 'barking' tics can be at any pitch – high, medium or low. They are sharp and short (often loud) sounds that frequently make other people jump. It can be a quick 'ooh', 'aah', 'oww', 'wah', 'pah', 'la', 'le', 'brrr', 'gaa' or one of the countless other monosyllabic sounds the human voice can make. Unlike a dog, Touretty 'barking' does not usually begin with a growl or end in an '–oof'. Touretty barking is never threatening. Yes, the occasional high-pitched Touretty bark could sort of resemble, say, a Yorkshire terrier's 'yap', just as the odd low-pitched vocal tic might resemble the grumble of a Rottweiler. On the whole, though, my 'barking' sounds nothing like a dog.

Now, this bog-standard Touretty barking is usually fairly 'motorised', much in the same way as the bodily tics. I tic verbally all day long. But not all of my vocal tics are very loud. With me, most of them are fairly low-key – continuous, but quiet. Usually, I make a sound (verbal tic) each time I exhale, so that means many thousands of vocal tics a day. Most last for half a second, although some 'choose' to last for two or three. Even though I generally find myself in a satisfying routine of verbal tics, I'll be forced at some point during each day to let rip with a really big, loud one, often very high-pitched and usually rather ear-splitting. I can only think that the reason for this is because most of the time I'm in 'quiet' verbal tic mode, or consciously trying to keep them as *sotto voce* as possible. In consequence, it seems that my brain gets to feel a little starved and proceeds to tweak my neurotransmitters into provoking a really large and ever-so-satisfying (for me and my brain) vocal tic. I can't begin to tell you how much of a release I feel, how relieved I am when I burst out with a wonderfully loud high note that most coloratura sopranos would die for. It's fantastic.

The problem with these vocal tics is the way that people treat me. If I'm in a shop browsing, I tend to get almost accusing looks from salespeople, who must somehow equate odd little sounds with shoplifting. Many a vigilant shopkeeper has stalked my every move, lest I pocket something when they're not looking. If I'm sitting quietly in a café – well, not always *so* quietly – minding my own business and reading, or even writing this very book, but making the inevitable little vocal tic each time I exhale, then people tend to stare. More often than not they change tables and move away. They seem to get scared for some strange reason. For goodness' sake, I'm only making little noises. Nothing about my image or behaviour is in any way threatening. OK, I'm talking about London and I suppose one can never really tell who the next rabid psychopath might be, but please, it's only me. I'm as gentle as it gets.

I once went into a church in London – the Brompton Oratory Church – to escape the hustle and bustle of nearby Knightsbridge, and I heard some strange noises. They were distinctive Touretty phonic tics. In fact, I actually had to stop and check myself over for fear that the noises I was hearing were coming from me, which for once they were not. My ear led me to the culprit, who was a boy of about thirteen. He was kneeling at a pew with his family and praying. His vocal tics were horrendous. Maybe the family was devoutly Catholic and was praying normally, or maybe the boy had been brought to the church in the hope that he might be purged of his symptoms. I didn't like to disturb them in their prayers so I never did get to find out, but I often wish I had spoken to them. Perhaps they, like so many thousands of people, had no idea that what the boy actually had was TS. What was interesting about the incident, and the reason I'm mentioning it now, is that I saw two well-heeled, middle-aged ladies scuttling rapidly towards the exit, rosaries in hand, and I overheard one of them say to the other, 'It's disgusting, bringing a boy like *that* into a church.' I can't tell you that I was in any way surprised by what I'd heard. If the boy had instead been, say, a disabled person in a wheelchair, a child with Down's syndrome or someone with some other easily identifiable illness or deformity, then I'm sure that the two ladies wouldn't have batted an eyelid. The fact that the boy was not able to fit into a convenient or obvious medical pigeon-hole rendered him an outcast, despite there obviously being something very wrong with him. Some people just cannot handle the different or the unknown. Not even in one of God's houses, it seems.

When I'm home alone I tend to let my vocal tics go crazy if that's what they want. I toot, bark, yell or whatever else I'm compelled to do. When I'm out and about, though, I do have to try with all my might to put a bit of a cap on the vocal tics, lest I generate too strong a reaction in other people. The perverse thing is that when I'm in a situation where vocal tics are utterly inappropriate – a hushed library, a church, a museum, an art gallery – then I absolutely have to make one of my really loud sounds. It's cruel that in the very situations where I just want to go unnoticed and pootle along insignificantly, my messed-up brain chemistry makes me do something that not only draws attention to me, but disapproval as well. I do consider myself lucky in being able to tone the verbal tics down a bit most of the time. I often remember the boy in the church and I thank my lucky stars that my vocal tics are not as severe as his were. I'm thankful, too, because if my toned-down version of vocalalia generates the disapproval, fear and suspicion that it already does, then I can't imagine what reactions I might provoke if I really had to let myself rip.

The trademark barking is not the whole story regarding vocal tics. Having to imitate sounds (technically called 'echolalia') also features in my dizzy world. With me, it's an abrupt or out-of-the-blue sound (usually high pitched, although not always) that does it. I *have* to imitate it exactly. Something in my brain clicks to life and sends me an order to imitate at all costs. It all happens so fast – within milliseconds probably – but I actually sense that I'm going to have to imitate the sound and know that, like any Touretty tic, bodily or otherwise, there is nothing I can do to avoid imitating it. A honk from a car horn might do it, the screech of breaks from a bus, the distant toot-toot of a train, a creaking door, the bleep of my computer when it boots up. And on and on. There are thousands of possibilities out there waiting to prompt me into imitation.

It can be very embarrassing, actually. And very frustrating because I'm a man and my voice is fundamentally low in pitch. Yes, a lot of my verbal tics naturally come out as falsetto high notes, but what happens if the sound that I am impelled to imitate exactly is too high for even *my* voice to ape? Well, like the Touretty touching, where I have to touch again and again until my brain lets me know that I've had a successful touch, it's exactly the same with imitating sounds. Luckily, I usually manage to hit the high note on my first attempt, but if it really is too high and on my first try both my brain and my ears tell me that I was way off, then I have to keep on trying until either by some miracle I do hit the note or my voice just gives in and refuses point-blank to try anymore. It's frustrating, painful and so perverse, and I often end up feeling such a failure. Imitative tics are yet another cruel strain of Tourette's. I remember when, as a child, if I was watching a television programme in which there was a train that tooted, then I'd have to imitate the train and go on imitating it again and again for an interminable period. We all thought it rather funny at the time, and it was too, but I'm grateful that nowadays my imitation is limited only to mirroring the sound I hear, just the once, not having to imitate it and continue doing so ad nauseam.

It is interesting that every medical professional specialising in TS I've met always clearly differentiates between bodily tics and verbal ones. The few books available in which TS is mentioned also seem to make the same distinction. I'm not quite sure why both researchers and medical professionals get it so wrong because I have absolutely no doubt that the verbal tics and the bodily ones are one and the same thing and are derived from exactly the same impulse within the Tourettist. True, some people may have verbal tics and no bodily tics, just as others will have exhausting bodily tics and no verbal ones, but full-blown Tourette's usually sees both the bodily tics and the verbal tics present.

Now, the reason that both tic forms should be considered one and the same is perfectly obvious to me. All of my vocal tics are accompanied, followed or preceded by a bodily tic. See. It's simple. I tic somewhere in my body as, or just before, or just after, I tic verbally. There is absolutely no time when I do one without the other. Both are preceded by that welling up from deep within – remember the blinking exercise? – and both invariably emerge in me from the same source, not, as we are led to believe, from different sources. For me a tic is most definitely bodily and verbal simultaneously.

Just as my bodily tics 'evolved' over the years – shaking, to nodding, to blinking, to clenching, etc – my vocal tics underwent a similar evolution. In truth, the tics, now that they have hopefully reached their full level of severity, just seem to be 'chosen' – picked out of a hat randomly by my brain according to its needs. Again, like the bodily tics, my repertoire of verbal tics contains a seemingly endless plethora of variations on a theme. As a child, when TS was taking its hold, I was a jumble of disorganised tics, but now my Touretty brain selects its various favourites. It equates choosing the particular tics it 'needs' each day, much in the same way as a child might choose sweeties in a sweet shop: today I'll have one of these, two of those and a whole box of that. A different selection of sweets every day for the spoilt child, a different choice of tics each day for the greedy Touretty brain.

Right now, and for the past year or so, in terms of its favourites, my brain has stayed with four distinct vocal tics. The first is the single medium-pitched 'hmmm' that I have to make almost every time I exhale – a 'hmmm' that must cause my vocal chords to vibrate so that I feel the vibration right through my head and all the way deep into the secret little sinus cavities around my face. The second is that wonderfully satisfying high-pitched loud yelp/bark that happens about thirty times a day, often catching even me by surprise. The third is awful. I'm forced to hyperventilate, something that's still classed as a vocal tic, even though it only concerns my breath. About once a minute (on average) I have to fill my lungs to what feels like capacity and then go on inhaling until I feel I'm about to burst. On exhalation, I then have to push all of the air out of my lungs and when they seem empty I must continue exhaling as though there is still air left inside. This hyperventilating thing is very motorised; I must perform both the excessive inhalations and exhalations to a steady pumping rhythm – usually at a pace of two pumps per second (I've timed it). On 'satisfactory' completion of air in and air out I must add a nice final touch to the whole procedure by making an 'ooh' sound that must – absolutely must – make the back of my throat and my epiglottis (I presume) vibrate. It's horrid. I feel I'm either about to explode from too much air in my lungs or pass out from having nothing in them at all.

Often, other people can hear my breathy little pumping sounds and, while most probably think I've got a bad dose of asthma, some give me very cautious or accusing looks, no doubt thinking that I'm some sort of sex pervert on a dirty little masturbatory high. I've been through this hyperventilating period many times in my life and have received all manner of reaction from others, but one particular memory of a reaction just won't leave me. I went to the Barbican Centre in London to hear a piano recital. There I was, alone and happily enjoying the music, when the woman sitting beside me pushed her face right up against mine and hissed loudly, 'You disgusting animal!' She then stood up, pushed past me and left noisily. I was mortified. I was devastated. As I sat in my seat, the silent screaming from inside me blocked out the music I had gone to hear: 'What am I? What *am* I?'

The last of my current verbal tics is bizarre. *Really* bizarre. You see, I blow raspberries! Go on, laugh. Please laugh. I do, and so does everyone who knows me. Most of these raspberries that I blow are tiny little ones – just a quick pursing of my lips and a tiny blow causing just the hint of a vibration and consequently a miniscule raspberry. I would say that for every five of my medium-pitched 'hmmm's each time I exhale, I have to blow one mini raspberry. It's so kinky, but again, ever so reassuring. The problem is that over a period of, say, every fifteen minutes, the mini raspberries will be getting marginally louder – it's a very gradual, almost imperceptible crescendo – resulting in one mother of a whopper raspberry that sounds very much like an imitation of exceedingly profound flatulence. Once the 'big one' has occurred, it's back to the minis again and the very odd cycle repeats itself.

Unfortunately, like the loud occasional yelp/bark thing that I have to make – the one that pops out unexpectedly – the quasi-flatulent raspberry is the same. I can't begin to tell you how embarrassing it is, or how unsuspecting people react. I'm sure they must regard me a bit of a nitwit if they actually see me pursing my lips and blowing a massive raspberry, or, if they don't actually see me doing it, but only *hear* it, then I guess they think I'm terribly impolite and in obvious need of medication. I can assure you again – I'm doing a lot of assuring in this book, but Tourettists are always *so* misunderstood – that I have absolutely no control over my vocal tics. *They* control me.

CHAPTER 7

INSTITUTIONAL BULLYING

When I was eleven my life changed and I embarked on a journey that would prove to be one of my most painful. I had to leave my friendly little primary school and move to a big secondary school, thus venturing head-on into a new world. Remember, I had not yet been diagnosed with Tourette's syndrome and, although I'd been seen by countless doctors, I still remained the boy with bad nerves, the boy with tics and twitches, the boy who touched things. The vocal tics had taken hold of me by then, so I was also the boy who made strange noises. I was literally thrown into a huge inner London school, and I was clearly very 'different'. In my old school people had become used to my Touretty ways. Everyone who knew me had become used to them. I'd had many friends and they'd all accepted me. Despite my glaring Tourettisms, my first year at secondary school passed more or less without incident. I was bright and clever. My tics and other Touretty things were violent, but somehow the other kids in my class didn't react badly towards me. I think they were all finding their feet in the big school too, so they weren't so eager to 'home in' on me just yet. Sure, a few people did mimic me and call me names, but on the whole I was able to shrug things off. A little harmless teasing never hurt anyone.

It was by a stroke of luck – I call it fate – that I discovered my vocation when I was all of eleven. I became obsessed with music and started piano lessons with a lady who lived a few houses along from ours. I was good at the piano. It was a strange turn of events, because my brother, Jeremy, had been a wonderful musician and the piano had been his passion too. But heroin had killed any chance Jeremy had of pursuing a musical career. In fact, my parents had been so devastated by his move away from music that they had long ago got rid of the family piano, as I suppose, to them, it stood as a constant reminder of how things used to be, of what might have been. As luck would have it (for me), my father was walking along our street one afternoon and saw an old upright piano sitting in someone's front garden. It had a sign on it that said, 'Good home wanted'. My parents couldn't resist it and engaged some friends into helping them trundle the battered old instrument along to our house. That piano was my saviour, and, in the years to come, would prove to be my only friend.

Suddenly I had a piano and, as if handed to me on a plate, I found love. School life continued, my tics remained brutal, home life was consumed by growing fears for Jeremy, but I didn't care. I practised that weathered old piano every moment that I could. I lived for my weekly lesson. I took my grade four after an unprecedented three months and grade five after six months. I lapped up music. I didn't realise then that it usually took people at least three or four years to reach the standard I had attained in a fraction of the time. I didn't know then that the piano would mould my whole future. I had no idea that it would be the cause of so much joy and heartbreak.

The strange thing surrounding my learning the piano was that when I played my tics almost seemed to disappear. It was like a miracle. I would tic, gyrate and verbally explode all day at school, get home exhausted from it all and run to the piano and play for as long as I could, not only because I loved the sounds that I was making, but primarily because when I played I didn't tic. I got time off from the ticcy normality that had become me.

Another year passed at school. I still ticced and I still played the piano. But all the beauty and respite I was experiencing within myself when I played the piano was gradually being smashed out of me by the bullying I suddenly began to endure at school. It was almost as if one day everyone was suddenly commanded to victimise me. I was mercilessly teased and mimicked for my tics and noises and touching, and I was ridiculed because the other kids had found out that I was good at the piano. It was evidently a girly or poofy thing to do. As the school year progressed, the bullying escalated. 'Don't talk to Blinker, he's obsessed with the piano,' or, 'Look, it's Noddy, the piano man,' or, 'Let's all watch the moron twitch,' or, 'Let's beat up the freak.' They aped me, they teased, they ganged up and they made my life hell.

And the teachers stayed silent.

I found solace each day when I returned home from the agony that was school – comfort and safety with my piano, which was a harsh contrast to the way things were panning out at school. In the classroom I was close to becoming the proverbial nervous wreck. In the playground I was punched, mimicked, laughed at, spat at, ambushed, kicked and often chased all the way home. I had only one or two friends, as few kids wanted to be associated with anyone who was the subject of so much ridicule. I was the freak and I was bullied for it. I was different and I was punished.

I often hear people talking about children and, inevitably, the phrase that pops up the most is, 'It's amazing just how cruel kids can be.' The expression usually makes me feel nauseous, for nausea is what I fought every day of my school life, right up until I was seventeen and left for good. I was a living example of their cruelty. I was being penalised daily for being different and I lived in fear. During school break times, when there were not so many teachers around, I used to hide in some secluded toilet, where more often than not I'd vomit from the fear of what they might do to me. I just couldn't cope with the teasing. Sometimes I would be found in my secluded toilet and, as well as physical abuse, they would roll about in hysterics as they saw me ticcing, shaking and hyperventilating myself into a state of frenzy. At some stage though, I made a pact with myself. No matter what they did to me, no matter how much they hurt me, no matter how spitefully or successfully they mimicked me, I would never let them see me cry. I would endure.

My teachers at school must have known that something was wrong, for not only did my school work deteriorate, but the boy, who, despite his tics, had entered the school so cheerfully three years before, was now timid, insular, uncom-municative and frightened. I actually think that they *did* notice the change in me, for they would have failed to be human had they not, but they *chose* to do nothing, they decided to take the easier approach of not 'getting involved'. I know that today schools are supposed to have very active anti-bullying policies, but my school, in the 1980s, maintained that it would not tolerate bullying either, so this wonderful anti-bullying thing is nothing new, even though we're sold it as though it is. The salient point is whether or not the teachers choose to act on the policies, as opposed to not bothering and thus having a quieter life. What good is policy without enforcement? For my part, I just couldn't understand why no one would step in and stop the pathological cruelty. For God's sake, it was almost institutional bullying. No action was taken, no support was given and no word of it was ever spoken. The teachers ignored me and the kids made my life a living nightmare.

But I didn't cry. I endured.

The years panned on, my tics remained as demonstrative as ever and I was still in love with the piano. I still gave my heart and soul to music. I remained the bullied and still managed not to cry. You might wonder why I never told my parents, why I never engaged their help. The answer was simple to me – if my parents had stepped in, if they had gone to the school, if they had tackled the problem, then I believed, like all bullied people, that things would only get worse. In fact, I was certain things would escalate. Also, I truly thought that if I were to tell my parents, their lives would completely fall to pieces. You see, things with Jeremy were deteriorating rapidly. He was spending time in and out of prison for dealing. The police were intermittently at our house looking for him. Drug dealers to whom he owed money began trying to terrorise my family.

Furthermore, Jeremy had become an active practitioner of black magic. Not the harmless, wand-waving, rabbit-out-of-a-hat, abracadabra stuff of simple conjuring magic, but heavy-duty, crypt-desecrating, black-mass, spiritually manipulative and soul-destroying evil. Alongside heroin, it had become his life. But for Jeremy, it wasn't a case of mild fascination, but more of an intellectual pursuit. He had long been mesmerised by the writings and practices of Aleister Crowley (1875–1947), author of a number of books on the occult and magic and someone who had enjoyed fame as 'the wickedest man in the world'. As well as being a wonderful musician, Jeremy had been one of these rare people whose intellect is frightening. Although his heroin addiction had, at times, rendered him the same as so many desperate junkies who walk the streets, his whole life had generally been consumed with the pursuit of knowledge as a means to bettering the soul. Although he became a drug addict in his teens, I believe that his use of heroin latterly became a way by which he believed he could transcend the plane of normality and reach a form of enlightenment, possibly much in the same way that the now notorious Dr Timothy Leary had recommended the use of LSD to his followers in the United States in the psychedelic 1960s. Also, the teachings of Aleister Crowley seemed to encourage this sort of practice, so the black magic and heroin went nicely together for Jeremy's purposes.

Crowley had set up an order for his followers, and an order loosely based on Crowley's original had been established internationally in the 1970s. Jeremy became the British director of this later order in the 1980s. Like all cults, the order required absolute obedience from its followers, and laid down extremely rigorous rules by which they should conduct their lives. However, Jeremy was eventually expelled from the group over a dispute relating to the copyright of some of Crowley's writings, which he had bought. Having offended the leader of the order, Jeremy was supposedly put on a 'death list' and was persecuted and threatened with murder from then on. Although the details have only filtered through to us over the years, it is quite clear that the cult really did actively persecute Jeremy, with the sole intention of making him fear for his life. As a result of further dispute with the publisher of Crowley's writings, Jeremy attempted to blow up their London warehouse and he was caught, convicted and sent to prison for two years.

Jeremy had lived with us intermittently since his twenties, at one stage living in our small summer house at the end of our garden. I remember that he barred us from entering it, but one day, when he was out, I managed to sneak in out of curiosity. I found myself surrounded by books on the occult, a suffocating smell of incense, magic symbols, a huge effigy of Crowley and walls covered with pentagrams. The reason that he was finally expelled from our home by my parents was due to his very disruptive influence on the family atmosphere, along with a suspicion of something rather more frightening. While he had been staying for a few days with my paternal grandmother, it is believed that he spiked her tea with the wildly hallucinogenic substance LSD. My grandmother, who had always been solidly down-to-earth and not one for flights of fancy, suddenly had an attack of crazy hallucinations. It began with her climbing onto the window ledge in her bedroom, proclaiming that she was about to fly off to somewhere better, and developed into a kind of nervous breakdown. She was unstable for many months, and would often interrupt conversations in order to converse with her late aunt, who she believed was sitting in a little glass box above the fireplace. This all did indeed sound similar to documented bad 'trips' with LSD and the long-term effects of the drug, so I can understand why my parents decided that Jeremy's presence in our home was just too dangerous. In fact, at one stage my parents suspected that Jeremy might have given me some sort of drug, which was causing my problems, but on investigation, they found that it was totally impossible in view of my symptoms.

The stress was killing my parents. The situation with Jeremy was desperate, and I didn't dare add to their misery by telling them of my utter unhappiness at school. I didn't want to. I hated to think of the consequences.

My parents never noticed any telltale signs of the bullied child because at home I *seemed* happy – all I did was spend time at the piano. I was, in a sense, despite all of my 'nerve' problems, a happy child at face value. I was no trouble, I was busy and I was sensitive. Perhaps my parents' vision was so clouded by despair for Jeremy that they didn't latch onto the fact that, like them, I too was dying inside, although for entirely different reasons. I do know with all my heart that it came as a massive shock to my parents when I recently told them some of what I'm now committing to paper. They really didn't know. They never saw.

My verbal tics became particularly bad at school. I was fourteen. There was no let-up from the constant bullying and still no concern from the teachers. What had began as small emotional scars were rapidly turning into great big open wounds. I had started to wear glasses and, as I made a loud verbal tic, I'd often shake my head so violently that my glasses would go flying. That, predictably, was the cause of much hilarity in the classroom. They barked in imitation of my Touretty noises and called me 'Doggy'. They snatched my glasses from me, hid them and shouted out, 'Go on, doggy. Go sniff for your glasses, you fucking blind bastard.' There was still no concern and no reaction from my teachers. None. Zero. I hated them all. I feared everyone. I lived in dread. But I still endured and never cried.

Through all the years of secondary school I never once saw a doctor about my 'nervous tics' and things. We had all given up seeking treatment as all prior routes had led to closed doors and phrases containing, 'grow out of it', 'nerves' and 'attention-seeking'. My father used to (and still does) give me head, neck and shoulder massages to help alleviate the pain, aching and stiffness from violent head-shaking, nodding and head-jerking. He was wonderfully patient with me and was always monitoring my behaviour in the hope of locating a cause for it. He taught me how to meditate, but it made me worse as the more relaxed I became, the less inhibited my tics would become. I took over-the-counter painkillers by the bucketful. I even had a go at being faith-healed.

My grandmother swore by the powers of a man called Jacob who visited her once a week and, with a laying-on of hands, helped her with general aches and pains. My parents were desperate enough to give anything a go, so I was deposited at my grandmother's home on the healing day. While Jacob was supposedly healing my grandmother I was told to wait in another room, but curiosity got the better of me and I managed to peep in to see what was going on. What

I saw blew me away. My grandmother was sitting on a wooden chair in the middle of the room with her eyes closed, and Jacob was standing in front of her with his hands hovering just a few centimetres above her ample bosom. He too had his eyes closed and was shuddering so hard it seemed like an electric current was being passed through him. He kept saying with a shaky and breathless voice, 'Can you feel it, can you *feel* it?' and my grandmother, who was also doing a bit of a shaky number herself, replied with an equally trembling voice, 'Yes, Jacob, I can, I *really* can.' It was most bizarre. When it came to my turn, though, I wasn't given anything like the same wobbly treatment – all Jacob did was hold his hands over my head and tell me to cleanse my spirit. Needless to say, it didn't cure me, so obviously my little spirit remained as impure as Jacob seemed to suspect.

We still had no name for my condition. No support. No idea that there were others going through exactly the same as I was. We had no choice but to accept.

To stop the bullying at school, I decided to engage the help of a higher authority. I started praying. Although I had been brought up in an entirely religious-free environment, I decided to turn to God. I wasn't sure if I actually believed in God or not, but I thought it was worth a try. I had nothing to lose. My pre-school prayer routine would start each night as I went to bed. I'd pray with all my might while clutching my deceased grandmother's rosary beads. 'Please God, help my nerves. Please take my tics away. Please let them stop hurting me. Please stop the bullying. Please stop their mocking. Please make me normal. Please help me. Please, please, please . . .' I would recite this prayer until I fell asleep and then continue in the morning as I made my way to school.

I wanted so much to believe that God would hear me. That if I asked enough He would help me. That prayer went on for years and years. But it was never answered.

The climax of those dreadful years at school – the event that still makes me go cold when I remember it – was when I had to endure victimisation not only from the whole class, but also from my teacher on that Wednesday during form period. It was a display of what I can only believe was pure evil. I'd contemplated trying to get my mother to allow me to stay home that day. I'd even considered protesting wildly at her decision that life should go on as normally as possible. You see my brother, Jeremy, had finally made the decision to end his beleaguered existence and had committed suicide the previous day. Family members and friends had converged on the house and, although most were trying to sleep when I left for school, I knew that, should I stay home, I would only be bombarded again with the words associated with death that had heavily permeated the atmosphere the previous night – funerals, post-mortems, coroner's inquests, coffins, flowers . . . In the end I had decided that it would probably best serve everyone if I just went to school, so I trundled off as normal. It was horribly coincidental that my brother's death and my own public undoing happened at the same time.

In class that afternoon, when the teacher sat and watched as the other kids in my form period jeered, spat at me, mocked and laughed, I was like a repugnant human exhibit in a Victorian circus sideshow. I was like a medieval village idiot in the stocks. And the teacher's joining in on the destruction of a scared little spirit made it a virtuosic study in humiliation and victimisation. It was utterly savage. It's an event from which I think I've never fully recovered, and I hardly think it's any wonder that I broke the pact I had made with myself and finally gave in and cried, even though I despised myself all the more for it. The sick thing was that they all enjoyed my tears. I really think it made them feel good about themselves. I knew that people could be cruel, I'd endured taunting, mocking and physical bullying for years, but that one merciless and concentrated dose of human poison was something that made me feel more utterly worthless, deficient and low than I'd ever imagined was possible.

When I got home that day, instead of sitting with my grieving family, I went and sat in my bedroom and begged the heavens to put me out of my misery and make me die too. I started to understand why Jeremy had been exhausted by life's journey and I began to respect him for having the courage to make an early exit. I did make one decision, though: I would never again pray for help. There simply wasn't any point.

Chapter 8

Numbers, Things, Details

I've been trying to describe to you the aspects of my Tourette's that you'd probably notice if you met me. But these symptoms, these trademarks, are not the whole story by far. To give you a vivid picture of the unseen and unnoticeable aspects of my Tourette's, the hidden and secret goings-on, I want to invite you into my head.

Numbers. Let's kick off with these. They feature enormously in my head and seem to be essential to my Touretty brain. Numbers do not consume me: I am consumed by *them.* Just like the bodily motor tics, the touching and the vocal tics, there is nothing I can do to stop my brain craving, registering and processing absolutely uninteresting and utterly useless numbers.

To try and show you how very different my brain is to yours, let me ask you a few simple questions: Do you know how many wheels a double-decker bus has got? Do you know how many windows your house or flat has? How many horizontal lines do you have on your forehead when you frown? The word Afghanistan has (no counting please) how many letters? How many pairs of shoes do you have? How many carriages did the last train that you took have and how many seats were in your carriage and how many were occupied when you alighted? Could you get all of those answers if you really, really thought about them? Probably not. In fact, I should hope that you couldn't. You would be somewhat odd if you could. Unfortunately, I know the answers to all of the above. My memory not only stores the information, this ever-so-uninteresting data, but actually adds to it and updates it on a daily, hourly, probably minutely basis, day in, day out, year after year.

In a café or wine bar, for example, I'll know how many bottles of alcohol are on the shelves behind the serving counter, which as it happens I have my back to, but which registered as I entered. I'll know how many tables there are, how many are occupied, how many floor staff are on duty, how many sugar cubes the lady at the next table put in her coffee, how many items are on the menu, how many acne spots our waitress has on her face, how many times the teenage girl at the next table says the infuriating word 'like'. I'll never relay these boring little details to you, or anyone else for that matter, and I'll never go home and jot down my numerical findings in a special notebook as a trainspotter might record train details. The data just 'went in' to my brain, was collected and processed, without me giving any of it a thought. It's almost marvellous, but it's not.

It doesn't stop there. My brain is not only constantly absorbing useless numerical data like a sponge does water, but it has the nerve to actually store it.

You will happily sit in a coffee shop and concentrate on

your coffee, a newspaper or on the person who is with you. Your concentration, or rather your broader vision of the details of your surroundings, will be, quite naturally, limited. You will be aware of *things*, people, etc in your rather blurred peripheral vision, but you will not be disturbed by them. You will not be bombarded by them.

Well, I unfortunately am numerically bombarded – assaulted by everything that is not only in my direct line of vision, but the peripheral stuff too. I'm not exaggerating, when I say that I'm assaulted by these numerical details I'm describing how it feels to me, as a Tourettist. Believe me, I don't want to be interacting with you while hearing 'twelve bottles of red wine, five women, eight men, three toddlers, two lumps of sugar, four employees, two cooks . . .' silently whispering to me from in my head, but I do. Like most Tourettisms, it's exhausting; I'll be constantly trying to filter the useless details out. They are not welcome in my head, but they remain there nonetheless.

What is curious is that numbers of things less than about thirty usually register immediately on sight. That is to say that I'm in no way actually consciously counting things up to that number. It just happens. The calculation is sort of automatic. Some little collection of brain cells, which could surely be getting on with something far more useful, made the calculation. I can live with this, despite the fact that those eccentric brain cells are constantly whispering data at me.

The problems occur when I'm looking at, or am aware of, things that number more than about thirty. My 'collector' brain cells get lazy then, and, instead of just getting on with their own counting, they employ me to do it for them. I could be in a crowded London shopping plaza, surrounded by a whole host of shops (not many of which interest me) and those numerically fascinated brain cells spot a counting opportunity – one that they can't handle alone – and force me to and take stock of my surroundings and manually count the number of shops, or benches, or rubbish bins, or people, or whatever. I try to do my best to ignore the need to count, but like the tics I described earlier, the need becomes stronger and stronger until it gets to be an absolute necessity. I am helpless to block out this greediest of cravings. I feel as though I'm almost floating around in a numerical nightmare. Large building facades with many windows are a particular problem for me. I'm literally forced to not only manually count the windows, but then to assess whether each floor has the same number of them. If it proves that they don't, then I have to make a mental note of which floors are different. The fact of the issue is that I'm never *not* counting. If Touretty obscenities are called coprolalia, and Touretty noises vocalalia, then this must surely be 'countalalia'.

Now this annoying counting thing doesn't only limit itself to external stimuli. My counting brain also logs and orders certain numerical combinations of some of my Touretty tics. It doesn't appear to be very interested in counting my run-of-the-mill head-shaking, nodding, clenching, hyperventilating, yelping, etc, but seems to pounce on certain particular ticcy things. Its favourites vary daily but usually involve the order to flex and let go of my calves, or roll my eyes painfully 360 degrees clockwise, or smash my teeth together a certain number of times, no more and no less. I don't know where the command to do these things comes from, all I know is that when I'm aware that I'm going to have to make certain tics, I know beforehand exactly how many I'm going to have to focus on executing. It must sound rather as though I actually choose to tic in these cases, but I really don't. There's no choice. I'm told to tic and that's that.

This counting lark often gets especially irritating when I'm in conversation with people. I find myself counting the number of times they say certain words. Again, I have no choice as to which word is chosen, and what usually happens is that I end up having to count very commonly occurring words, like 'it', 'and' or 'me', words that occur almost innumerably (but not to me) when people chat. If only my brain would choose a word like, say, 'obsequious', then I wouldn't have the running count endlessly going on, as people tend not to use that particular word very often.

Another greedy compartment of my brain seems to force me to examine *things*. It has to know exactly what is what and what is where. I know that everyone is vaguely aware of the things around them, but I am bombarded with close-ups. Wherever I go, my brain is literally flashing almost larger-than-life images of things in front of my eyes, so I not only know what the thing is, but am also aware of *where* it is in relation to all the other things around it. It's almost as though my brain is conducting an inventory of things wherever I am.

These things that burst into my awareness are not just the obvious ones. An ordinary room, for example, might contain a sofa, some chairs, a television, books, rugs and paintings. Most people will not notice every little ornament on the mantelpiece, or the names of the authors of the books, or which magazines you have stashed under your coffee table. People might see these things subconsciously, but they won't actively focus on them, categorise them and store the images, their details and their locations. I'll not only some-how have to process all the information being thrown at me, but I'll end up remembering it forever.

This same awareness occurs with people, too. I tend to stash away the details of what people are wearing, or holding, or doing, and have the information to hand years later. I also remember aspects of people's situations. I may meet someone once and chat for five minutes, but I'll remember everything they've told me, right down to the last detail. I often startle people I met years ago by telling them the exact date we previously met, what they were wearing and all about everything they happened to have said to me. Now these people usually mean almost nothing to me, play no part in my life and were to all intents and purposes just breezy five-minute chatty encounters. I'm sure the brain isn't meant to remember the details of almost everyone we meet. It must surely have all manner of little filters operating that sift out what is important and what really is not. I think that in my case, my brain is not filtering information out, but sucking it in, like a greedy vacuum cleaner. And it isn't particular about what it sucks in, either. It seems that everything and anyone will do: all welcome, numbers relished, personal details craved. This kind of strange memory syndrome is sometimes referred to, in a non-Tourette's context, as an 'eidetic' mem-ory or total recall, and it is considered a gift. Well, in terms of the piano I do see it as a gift, but in everyday living? It's just bloody annoying.

Sometimes it all gets just too stressful. Things around me in certain situations become too much for me to handle. You see, my brain doesn't seem to actually care about me, the per-son. As I keep saying, it's a greedy, selfish, Touretty brain. It wants and wants and wants, and then wants more. Super-markets, to take one common example, are hell on earth for me. So many aisles and shelves and stacks and various products, and, usually, so many people. I have to count, count, count, things, things and more things. People zoom in and out of my focus, one after another after another, with warped and distorted faces. Their voices seem to blast towards me as I become acutely sensitive to every little sound. It's like the most horrific psychological thriller, with the best special effects ever, except that I'm the one really living it. I just can't switch it off and, as the plot thickens, I find there's no way out. I want to scream 'HELP!' I want to drop everything and run, but I can't. And while all these wonderful special effects are playing out, I'm ticcing and hyperventilating and touching and vocally ticcing. It's shattering. For me, your world can be terrifying.

CHAPTER 9

TOUCH HEAVEN

So, I was a teenager with enough emotional baggage to bring down a 747. I had been crushed by teachers and pupils alike. I lived my life in fear, and where before I had been fuelled by an ability, an absolute obsession to endure, I was now left with not even that. My final school years dragged out miserably, but it was interesting that the bullying almost ceased completely after that huge and awful spectacle of me breaking down and being broken, which had been so thoroughly enjoyed by everyone. In retrospect it seems that this act of public humiliation rendered me of no further interest. There was nothing more they could do to me, you see. Their years of tormenting me had given them the one final kick that they had so long desired, and to cap it all I had been broken officially, in the sense that a teacher, into whose care we had been entrusted, had overseen, participated in and validated the proceedings, as though she had been a Roman senator watching a Christian being fed to the lions in an arena. I was a nothing.

I'm certain that my classmates, should they ever have the cause to remember me, will only remember the ugly, scared guy who twitched, made animal noises and provided so much entertainment. I know enough about life now to be able to at least *try* to understand why they made me their victim and human punchbag. I suppose it all boils down to the fact that they were finding their own feet in the big world as young adults and, like all adolescents, they were probably riddled with their own insecurities. The last thing they would ever have wanted was to draw attention to *themselves*, so what better way to deflect attention than by ganging together to focus on someone else, a weaker someone, a boy who wore his glaring defects and insecurities like a bright flashing sign attached to his head saying, 'victimise me'. Or maybe bad luck simply placed me in the close proximity of fundamentally cruel people. I have a feeling that the truth lay somewhere between the two, but, whatever the case, I was left as nothing more than damaged goods. The freak. The boy with the emotional wounds that would take decades to heal. All these years later I can still hear their mocking voices and see their twisted faces glowing with hatred and invigorated with victorious glee. Accuse me of holding a grudge if you wish, but I'm afraid I'm nowhere near the point of being able to forgive, let alone forget, clichéd as that may sound.

So the bullying ceased and I served out my remaining school years in a state of acceptance, rather like, I suppose, a victim of severe torture who realises that nothing more can be done to hurt him.

However, what my contemporaries never saw was my other personality. As the energy was draining from me at school, so it was fuelling the growth of the real me, the confident me, the strong and musical me. As one aspect of me died, the other learned to live. I was obsessed and consumed beyond measure with music. I heard it constantly in my head and I became able to block out the ugliest situation by mentally tuning in to beautiful sounds. To hell with school work, I now spent every possible moment locked away in what was called our 'music room'. There I would practise furiously for hours on end, never tiring and never ceasing in my quest to become better and better. And I did improve. Soon, the old battered piano that had been my saviour was deemed not good enough for me. My parents bought me a grand piano and I would sit at it, learning my pieces, imagining that I was a great concert pianist performing to an applauding audience. I spent all my pocket money on records – Beethoven, Brahms, Rachmaninoff and on and on – and I would listen again and again to each until I knew every nuance off by heart, every miniscule detail and every turn of phrase. Then I would play the recording at full volume and sit at my piano miming, imagining that it was me playing so wonderfully.

I had been having lessons with a local, much-respected teacher, and she encouraged me to explore harder and more complex repertoire. I dedicated my whole life to each piece, and found myself in a wonderful and private heaven, one in which I could escape not only my fears and emotional wounds, but also my tics, jumping, nodding, noises and hyperventilating. I was able to develop the musical me while having time off from what I now know was the Touretty me. Having said that, I must explain that while I was indeed escaping the exhausting Tourettisms, I know that I was simultaneously feeding and fuelling my Tourette's by giving it a thing it so craved: touch. The piano appealed to my fingers. You will remember how specifically, how methodically and how accurately I am compelled to touch things. The piano provided touch heaven for me – eighty-eight keys all sitting and waiting for my needy little fingers. The specific force of touch, or the weight behind each finger required in a successful Touretty touch, the touch that rendered so much of my life a ritualistic 'touch-mare', was now deployed on each note of each piece that I played. One of the main problems that anyone learning the piano must overcome has to do with brain-to-finger connection – the brain instructing the fingers to play a particular note, or notes, with the right pressure, at the right time. This connection usually develops slowly and it often takes years of repetitive practice to make the fingers react *with* the brain and not lag *behind* it. With me, because I had spent so many years touching things in a specific way, my brain–finger connection was super fast. It was a blessing. I learnt piano repertoire at lightning speed and was able to play it almost uncannily accurately. I found that I could read harder and harder pieces on sight. While most piano students at my level were working on technical exercises and playing scales, I was learning one piece after another and never once having to slog away with technique-strengthening exercises, for my technique was completely natural and inbuilt, courtesy of Touchy Tourette's.

Memory, or remembering pieces, causes pianists the most anxiety, as there is always the possibility of forgetting how a piece goes mid-performance. My memory, thankfully, lapped up every detail of the pieces I played. My apparently superhuman ability to store details and never forget made me certain that I had not only my Touretty fingers to rely on to play the notes with perfect accuracy, but the extra advantage of knowing that I would never forget a piece halfway through. My brain had everything under control, processed, logged, at hand at any time, any day. I didn't realise then what was going on, in fact, I assumed that everyone's brain must be like my own. I was able to play pieces without a thought, and if I was to actually 'think' while playing I could see the notes on the pages with my mind's eye and follow their progression as the music went along, turning the pages as the music went forward, even seeing the page numbers.

Becoming so involved in music led me to cultivate the solitary existence, to which I'd already been sentenced by my Tourette's, and turn it into my very own secret and safe haven. While kids of my age were out socialising, or doing whatever it is they did (I never found out), I was permanently locked away in my own private and magical world of sound and touch. Since the bullying at school had ceased, I suppose that you might imagine that I felt more comfortable in the school environment. But it was not the case. You see, I know *now* that the bullying most definitely did stop, I can even have a stab at understanding *why* it stopped. But at the time, I had no idea that it had indeed ended. I just felt relieved at each day that passed without being bullied, but still lived in fear of the following day.

I was so overly sensitised, so utterly derelict by school, that I never once dared let my new-found confidence in myself as a musician filter through into a world where it would not be appreciated – the last thing on earth I wanted to do was draw attention to myself. I was two distinct people – bursting with excitement and enthusiasm for music at home and petrified and ignored at school. I was very confused by the fact that my life, and indeed my personality, was so black and white. The only constants were my tics and yelping and touching and counting and eye-rolling and jerking, etc.

At home, apart from when I was in my music room, my Tourettisms still caused concern, still upset the status quo, and still left me physically shattered. Susanna, who spent periods living at home as well as away, still regarded me as an attention-seeking weakling. There seemed to be real resentment there. Far from seeing me as a little brother with obvious and mega problems, she actually still believed that I was putting on an act. I couldn't for the life of me understand why she was so hostile and sometimes even downright nasty. I knew I was putting on no act. She must have known that no one could possibly keep up such a per-formance year in, year out, day in, day out. If I'd really been acting I should have been awarded multiple Oscars, includ-ing one for sheer stamina. Moreover, Susanna was fit and dazzling, and had a wealth of suitably sporty and gorgeous friends, who all had much more important things to do with their time than pay attention to a bespectacled little thing like me. I did actually like one of Susanna's friends, she was the only one who was ever rather nice to me, but I went right off her when, one Saturday evening, after she and Susanna had been getting ready all afternoon for a big night out, she looked at me in utter horror and said, 'My God. It's Saturday night and you're staying in? Don't you have any friends?' I really didn't know what to say, so Susanna answered for me. '*Him* going out? You must be kidding!' It was said in such a derogatory fashion, as though I was the most hideous crea-ture on earth and shouldn't ever be allowed out. Although I knew that on that particular Saturday night, and countless others before and after, I had a wonderful time playing the piano and listening to music alone, I suppose deep down I would loved to have gone somewhere. I saw Susanna as so strong and popular and I desperately wanted to be her friend, and for her to be mine, but I knew I was the freak, and an ugly embarrassment.

The fact that I began living for, and excelling at, music seemed to ruffle Susanna's feathers almost as much as my 'acting' did. She labelled me a snob because I loved classical music. I was now an attention-seeking elitist. She said I was trying to be like Jeremy (God forbid!) and would never be as good a pianist as he had been. All I wanted was for her to have some time for me, to give me some of her astonishing strength, some of her physical perfection, some of her confidence. But it was not to be for many years.

I don't think a day went by when my parents didn't worry about my 'nerves'. Despite the fact that they had absolutely no idea of my other life at school, they became overly protective. Since Jeremy's suicide, they were naturally oversensitive themselves. My mother especially became terrified for me, no doubt imagining how, with my violent tics, I would fare in the real world. Little did she know that I already had a vivid, all too literal idea of how I would fare. I suppose that, for want of a better expression, my mother smothered me, wrapped me in cotton wool and overindulged me. No pressure was put on me to do anything. I was never told to work at the piano and I was never forced to do school work. An image of a spoilt child springs to mind, but that image would not fit the way things were. I was simply allowed to live peacefully in my private world of music and Tourette's syndrome. I had no real needs, save being left to get on with whatever gave me calm and pleasure and, despite the violence of my tics, I was not a needy boy. My parents had long accepted that that was how I was. There was nothing to be done. That I was so into my music was a source of relief to them, for Jeremy had, at the same age, abandoned his music entirely and already taken his first few steps down a path that would end in tragedy.

Jeremy's suicide, rather than pulling my parents together, had thrown them apart. My father, a quiet and private person at the best of times, became more private. His days were spent at work and his evenings alone, playing the guitar or playing chess. My mother, in complete contrast, became ever more sociable and gregarious. She's quite a phenomenon in herself, my mother. She's a woman of extremes. It's all *and* nothing with her. She warded off the daily emotional blows as she witnessed Jeremy's ruin with a strength I could never have imagined she possessed. She could have gained success and recognition as a writer, but she closed her notebook and never put pen to paper again. Her last piece of writing was a potent article for the *Guardian* about death, heroin and emotional destruction, written in the weeks following Jeremy's suicide. It was reprinted in a number of other publications such was its power, but after that, she claimed she had nothing more to say.

Yoga, people and politics became my mother's pastimes. I would frequently emerge from the music room, go looking for my mother and find her standing on her head in the middle of her bedroom floor, or on all fours, back arched, in the 'cat' position. Other times she would be happily humming along in her own world, aided by a good many gin and tonics on an empty stomach, empty because she was so figure conscious that most of the time she barely ate. Sometimes I'd emerge to find her in the lounge debating furiously with some of her Labour Party cronies – she'd had great political aspirations at one point, but her frequent attendance at meetings caused trouble with my father and after a few years she gave it all up completely.

My mother had, and still has, a curious personality that attracts people who are needy. It must be her warmth and positive outlook, but we would often have to endure all kinds of emotionally crippled people in our home day after day. Some of them, no doubt, had real problems of their own, but others, almost certainly, were just common garden-variety moaners, people who would grouch over life, whatever their circumstances. Maybe because these people saw so much misery in our home they felt that they could unleash their own in a 'safe', similar environment, or perhaps the ener-gies of our home pulled the misery out of them. Whatever the case, we were always too polite to burden them with our problems, not that we wanted to, and, on the whole, we listened patiently to their accounts of woe and made all the right sympathetic noises. Perhaps that's why they kept on coming back. There was always some poor soul sitting there, droning on and on. More often than not, I was in a terribly violent Touretty state, unable to keep still (or silent) and pale with exhaustion, my parents were demolished by Jeremy's death, Susanna was dealing with all number of her own issues, and these negative wrecks would have the audacity to tell us how miserable *their* lives were. To this day I have a personal phobia of 'needy' people and I tend to avoid them like the plague. I just don't do emotional wrecks. I can't.

CHAPTER 10

DETECTIVE WORK

We lived in an enormous, rambling Victorian London house, with its rooms scattered over many floors. It was amazing just how much could actually go on in that house, incredible how much one could do, without anyone else ever knowing. We were all up to our ears in our own peculiar little existences, but we never got in each other's way. The house gave each of us a great deal of privacy, something that I particularly valued, not only because of my music, but also because I hated anyone seeing me at my Touretty worst.

My secluded music room stood not only as a place where I could practise my piano and listen to records without ever disturbing anyone, but it also stood as my safe space, where I was able to let rip with some of my most extreme Tourettisms. I could yelp, bark, blow enormous raspberries, jump in the air, shake my head – or any part of me – as violently as I needed and never be in fear of someone seeing, or even hearing. Outside my music room I would try, with all my might, to stifle, or at least take the excessive edge off, my tics. I knew that my 'nerves' were still a source of anguish to my parents and I couldn't bear watching them watching me, fighting their own inner torment that stemmed from being unable to help. They were powerless, and I neither wanted them, nor anyone else who happened to be around, to see me so out of control.

It was around this time – I was fifteen – that I began asking questions. Maybe some place deep inside of me just got curious, or maybe it was a natural part of the growing up process, but I started quizzing my parents about my 'bad nerves'. For nine years we had all just let them be. Doctors had been seen, their opinions had been weighed up and ultimately rejected, but, on the whole, we had all just accepted that, whatever it was I had, the only solution was to let it run its course. After all, there was nothing life-threatening about it. The issue for me had never been why do I do it, but why do I *have* to do it? That was the enigma. It was strange, because as I started my little investigation, I began to take a different view of the way I was. I spoke endlessly with my parents about how it all started. I quizzed them on the details, on any circumstances I might have forgotten. We really tried to analyse why I ticced and did all my weird things, or, rather, what was *making* me behave in that way. I suppose for my parents, they were covering old ground, but for me, it was self-exploration. It was no longer good enough for me to say, 'I have to do it'. I wanted to know more. I wanted some answers.

I seemed to remember that Jeremy had indeed had various twitches and a few odd, almost involuntary, movements. I talked to my parents about this memory and they verified that he did have some obvious, rather uncontrolled tics and movements. But were his the same as mine, or, rather, did they stem from the same source? I didn't know and I couldn't dig too greatly because my parents just weren't able to talk much about Jeremy, and I couldn't blame them for that. But one thing I did manage to get from them was that he had been similar to me on two clear counts: he had (occasionally) shaken his head violently and rolled his eyes back hard in their sockets and, secondly, he was, or rather had been, absolutely involved mentally and physically in music. It was obvious that there were at least tenuous similarities between me and Jeremy, but there were also many differences. For me, the major difference, as far as I could ascertain, was that his tics did not start when he was seven. But, I wondered, did 'bad nerves' in siblings have to begin at a certain age? I was stabbing in the dark. Whatever age Jeremy had developed his tics remained obscured by the gruesome events that would eventually culminate in him taking his own life.

For the time being, Jeremy was a dead end, quite literally. So I looked at Susanna and examined her closely. I wanted to see some similarity between us and I desperately needed to see 'bad nerves' peeping through her immaculate exterior. Susanna must have been under my diligent scrutiny for about a week, during which I was on the lookout for any little twitch, grimace, tic or involuntary movement, any extra sound, or any odd touching. But my efforts were in vain. Susanna was clean, and, in any case, I really believed that she was so physically perfect, so confident and so vivacious, that it would have been next to impossible for her to be flawed like me.

I stumbled on a major clue, or one that I believed was such, when I overheard my mother telling a group of her political cronies that her mother had suffered terribly from

St Vitus' dance when she was a child. Later that evening, I asked my mother what particular dance Granny had. I had only vague memories of my mother's mother, as she lived in South Africa, which is where my mother was born, but I couldn't for the life of me remember her dancing in any of them. My mother explained that my grandmother had suffered all of her life with a 'terrible nervous condition', one that made her click her chin up and down (warm . . .), jerk her limbs about (warmer still . . .) and make seemingly involuntary movements (Bingo!).

'But that's exactly what I do,' I said to my mother.

'Yes, but Granny's was somehow different,' she explained. 'It was less violent and more nervous.'

I couldn't believe what I was hearing. That just didn't make sense.

But my mother went on to categorically assure me that there was no way I had St Vitus' dance.

And then she dropped the bombshell.

'Even if you did have it,' she said, 'I'd never let them treat you for it. They tortured Granny.'

Tortured Granny?

This was all news to me, and I sat in stunned awe as my mother explained.

All through her childhood, and for a great deal of her adult life, help from the medical profession had been sought for my grandmother's involuntary movements. Apparently, as a child, having been mercilessly teased by other children (I could relate to that) and castigated by her family for pulling awful faces and jerking her body, she had been taken to a physician, who said that, without a shadow of a doubt, she was displaying the signs of something called St Vitus' dance, or Sydenham's chorea. The treatment, my mother said, had not consisted of drugs but was of a far more physical nature. It had consisted of wrapping her body in blankets, alternating between ones taken from a bucket of ice and others taken directly from a tub of scalding water. This was supposed to somehow 'shock' the body into normalising itself. This undoubtedly excruciatingly painful treatment had gone on for ages.

That sounded pretty much like torture to me, and made the Valium I had been prescribed look like a golden nugget in comparison.

I spoke to my mother endlessly about my grandmother's symptoms – how similar to mine they had been, when exactly they had started, did the blanket torture help, did she make noises too and did she touch things?

However I approached it, though, my mother remained firm in her comparative diagnosis. I did not have St Vitus' dance. The doctors would have spotted it, and, even if they had, there would be no blanket baths for me. It was almost as if my mother knew that I *did* have St Vitus' dance, but refused to admit it even to herself, for fear that I would be treated in the same way as her mother had been. I, on the other hand, silently rejoiced. I had a name for my condition, or at least one that really sounded feasible. I vaguely knew what it was. I was the same as Granny. I never voiced all of this to my mother, of course, but knowing was enough for me.

It was at this time that my piano playing suddenly improved beyond all expectation. I was propelled and driven even more into my world of piano, touching, notes, sound and beauty. I'd met a boy, through one of my mother's many friends, who attended one of the London music colleges each Saturday, where he was, according to his mother, given 'the best musical education in the country'. And to top it all, it was free because the local council paid the tuition fees. Well, to me, this news was earth-shattering. I wanted to go to music college on Saturday mornings, too. I had to.

I asked my parents what they thought of the idea, and they said that it might be a great move if the fees were indeed paid by the local authorities, but probably not possible if they were not. But I couldn't let it go and became so obsessed with the idea that the following Monday I feigned a sore throat and procured the day off school. As soon as the house was empty, I phoned our local authority music advisor and pleaded my case. She turned out to be very helpful and enthusiastic, and had actually heard of me, apparently from my piano teacher, with whom she was friends. But the auditions at the music colleges, she said, had taken place months ago and there was no way I'd get a place in any of them for the following academic year, so I should hold on and wait it out.

I was so disappointed I could have cried. I'd had visions of being taught by great musicians, images of going off each Saturday to a real music college where I would meet other people just as in to music as I was. I became stubborn. I decided to phone the music colleges directly and ask if there was some way that I could be considered for a place. The first two reaffirmed what I had already been told. I was too late. My last hope was with the Royal College of Music, a college I had deliberately not phoned because I had always been told that it was the best of the colleges and that its standards were seriously high. I was so nervous when I phoned the Royal College, my hands were shaking and my voice quivered as I asked someone in the Junior Department if I was too late to be considered. I was stunned by the answer. The helpful lady said that they were full for the following year, but that they often made exceptions in special circumstances, if the standard of the applicant was high enough. She sounded a bit doubtful when I told her that I'd only been playing the piano for four years, but nonetheless invited me along to audition that very week. As I hung up the phone I nearly wet myself with excitement. The thought of going to the renowned Royal College of Music, for an audition they were holding just for me, was almost more than I could cope with. I ran to my piano, hooting, yelping, nodding and ticcing as I went, and started choosing the pieces I would play to them.

I told my parents what I'd done, of my little triumph, and my mother phoned our local authority to see whether they would pay the fees if I was accepted. Apparently they made all the right noises, so off I went that Thursday to the RCM and, for the first time in my life, passed through its imposing doors. What happened next was like a dream. I was ushered into a room and asked to wait until I was called. For ten minutes I sat there, not thinking about the pieces I was about to perform, but willing my tics to go away and not let me down in something I needed so much. As I sat, stifling my tics, I was engulfed in an absorbing sound world that was delicious beyond words. I was assaulted by a blur of music, a magnificent discord of instruments playing all at once – a cello there, a violin here, a piano cascading, the drone of distant lectures, the forces of an orchestra playing Brahms. I knew I had found my home. There, and only there, was where I wanted to be. I can't really recall much about the actual audition, but I remember being startled, dwarfed, in fact, by the size of the piano I had to play, and I remember that when I started to play it made a sound so sublime that I could have wept. Suddenly there was an almost deafening silence. I had played my two pieces and there was a momentary pause. I looked at my auditioners – there were four – and they were all beaming at me. They asked me why I wanted to study at the RCM, and I still remember my reply. 'Because I need to. I *have* to.' The next comment from them knocked me for six. 'You play absolutely beautifully. Who do you want to study with?'

My dream had come true, and a few months later, I started attending the RCM on Saturdays. I was allocated a teacher and I worked for him as though my whole existence depended on his approval. All I could think about were my piano lessons and the music I was learning and, in my mind, living and breathing.

As my miserable weeks at school seemed to go on forever, I would be thinking of one thing, and one thing only: Saturday. I saw Saturdays as my prize for living in fear all week. Saturday was my delicious reward. Saturday was all that counted.

At sixteen, my entire Touretty repertoire of tics, noises, thoughts, desires and touching had fully matured and developed. In the years to come there would be no startling new items added to my already exhaustive list of 'bad nerve' symptoms, or what I secretly believed were symptoms of St Vitus' dance. My parents still worried – I could see it in their faces – but they were heartened by the new-found confidence I was developing, since starting at the RCM Junior Department.

I started playing truant from school, or bunking off, as it was called. I would miss classes, whole afternoons, whole days sometimes, to stay at home working at the piano, getting better and better. My parents had no idea that I was truanting and the school never once tackled them, or even me, about my absence. At school, I was a nobody and so unregarded by everyone that it was of no interest whether I was there or not. Instead of the bullying I was ignored. In fact, I was so ignored that I sometimes wondered if I was invisible. My classmates had all grown up a little and I suppose the attraction of bullying the already-broken freak had lost its appeal, especially when in direct competition with sexual attraction. Their hormones were going crazy, and I suppose all they thought about was sex. Why pick on me when probing tongues and willing, open mouths were more exciting? For me, it all seemed so disgusting. They were like animals, but I knew that anyway. Furthermore, I didn't see the appeal of the girls around me, and, although that gave me slight pause for thought, I didn't dwell on it too hard because there were so many other things occupying me. In any case, I had no intention of lusting after anyone, not that anyone would have been seen with me. I was too ugly. I felt so ugly. All I cared about was music.

The months flew by and suddenly I had been attending the RCM Junior Department for a whole year. What's more, I had more friends from those single Saturdays than I had ever had in my whole life. I was involved in so much music-making on those cherished Saturdays, and I was suddenly not the freak. Bullying was an impossibility in such an environment. The other kids saw past my tics, perhaps were even oblivious to them, and treated me as an equal, as another musician – Nick the pianist, Nick the human being.

For the first time in my life I felt safe.

Chapter 11

A Brain in Conflict

In order to try to demonstrate what really goes on inside my head, I had to ask other people what was going on in theirs. The result showed me that my brain is doing extremely different things to most people's.

I really can't give you a biological explanation of what's going on – this chemical does that, to those cells, which in turn stimulate these transmitters, etc. But if I had to sum up the essence of what I'm about to try and explain, I would say that in my brain my thoughts, my desires and my emotions are all racing about furiously and going in whichever direction they please, all bumping into one another and all running with their engines at full throttle.

Hidden thoughts and a running commentary: we all have these. Our brains never really stop. You're doing one thing and, suddenly, out of the blue, another totally unconnected thought pops into your head. You don't know why, it just did. You also chat away to yourself in your head, although most of the time you aren't particularly aware of this one-sided little chat that is going on, as you are usually preoccupied with whatever you're doing. This chat thing is usually labelled 'thinking'. Shopping lists probably play themselves in your head, a reminder to set the video recorder for a television programme, thoughts about friends and family, ideas about how to spend your weekend, work-related things, sexual and lusty thoughts. We all have them.

So what about the desire to spit into some people's faces – one of their eyes, to be precise? I don't suppose you have that too. I hope you don't, because I know how infuriating and frustrating that particular desire is.

I want to spit in some people's eyes. *Want* to do it, that is. Sometimes. It's quite a hideous thought really, quite disgusting. But I'm not saying that I do spit at people. I just want to. I can't help it.

This spitting thing ('spitalalia', perhaps?) thankfully isn't something I'm actually forced to do. It's not a compulsion and it's definitely not a kinky obsession or an obsessive thought. It's not as a result of some inner hatred towards anyone, nor is it something I want to do to show how disgusting I think someone is, or for that matter to show how disgusting I am. Nothing of the kind. Simply put, I have a desire to spit in the eye (usually the left one) of only a miniscule number of people. There is nothing special about these people, liking them or disliking them doesn't enter into the quirky equation, there's never anything distinctive about their left eye that would render it particularly spit-worthy and there is no connecting or common feature among these people other than my desire to spit at them. I do think that somewhere along my muddled neurotransmitter line this spitting thing might somehow be related to the raspberry-blowing vocal tic. I do sometimes spit a lot as I'm walking along the street, but that's usually to try to disguise – or at least give some validity to – blowing a raspberry. But the actual desire to spit *at* someone leaves me more than slightly baffled. It doesn't *feel* like another motor tic because it involves my mouth.

I'm afraid I really just don't know where this horrible desire originates in my brain. All I know is that I can go days, weeks or even months on end without giving spitting in someone's eye so much as a thought, and then, suddenly, someone tickles my eye-spitting fancy and that's it. It can be anyone. However, what I do know is that if I were to meet you and *not* have the desire to spit in your left eye, then that's how it would stay. I wouldn't one day suddenly change and want to spit at you. It's black and white. Luckily, there aren't many people who set off my spit-in-the-eye alarms, but being around such people is incredibly frustrating. The thought keeps nagging at me and whispering tempting suggestions, 'Wow, look at that lovely round eye, see how it moves. If only you could just take aim and . . .' It's so annoying. Then the temptation becomes more of a need. 'Go on, you can feel yourself salivating. Now, all you have to do is . . .' Then it gets demanding and dictatorial. 'Spit! Go on, do it . . . NOW!' But I know I can't. I do everything I can to try and avoid looking at the eye that seems to look back at me like a waiting target. Everything is screaming at me to do it, but I – me the person – I don't want to. I won't. It's just too awful.

It's not only people I actually know, or am introduced to, who get me going. This only happens rarely, but occasionally my saliva ducts get excited by people I don't know at all. One example is a girl of about twenty who works in my local supermarket at one of the many checkouts. Supermarkets make me busy at the best of times, but my local one takes on a new dimension entirely if I amble in to do my shopping and see this particular girl perched at her till. My saliva ducts go berserk and I fly around like a man possessed, driven by one desire and one desire only, that of being served by the unsuspecting girl, quietly salivating and taking mental aim at her big, blue left eye and . . . and then, of course, not being able to do it, because every ounce of decency overcomes the wicked whisperings in my head.

The spitting is just one of the things that can, and sometimes does, cause my brain to play a little script to me. Insulting people, or rather mentally insulting them, is far more common. It's not that I'm a vindictive person by nature, quite the contrary, I hope. Before I open a particular can of worms that says that all Tourettists swear and insult people, suffer from Potty Mouth Tourette's, or coprolalia, let me reiterate that I'm not badly afflicted in this way. I do, however, obviously have a very mild version of it. I don't swear again and again out loud, nor do I think expletives in a motorised way, but I do sometimes severely and repeatedly insult people in my head. Now this isn't the same as you saying silently to yourself, 'Silly old cow,' when the shop assistant gives you attitude. It's not like you saying, 'Fuck you', or worse, when you run for the bus, only to have the driver close the doors in your face as you get to it. My insults are rarely spoken aloud, but run a usually very large and incredibly detailed (abusive) script in my head, while I'm actually standing next to, or even talking to, my particular victim. What happens in my head often seems to bear no relation to the situation I'm in. I can be with someone with whom I'm close, or simply with a complete stranger. The person I'm with has probably not offended me in any way, but, unexpectedly, my brain will start nagging at me and yelling a script at me that is sometimes very hard to block out. Here's an example: Recently, I popped into my local bookshop and asked the man behind the counter if he had any books in stock on Tourette's syndrome.

He stared blankly back and said, 'No we don't,' in a flat and unenthusiastic tone.

The script started: 'What do you mean? You have an encyclopaedic knowledge of all your books and know for a fact that there's not one on TS?' my head said.

My voice said, 'But do you actually know what TS is?'

He said, 'No,' plain and simple.

My head said, 'If you don't bloody well know what it is, then how can you possibly say you have no book on it?'

I said, 'Well, it's a neurological syndrome . . .'

'. . . asshole!' my head added.

He said, 'Look over there, under self-help.'

My head said, 'Look, you lazy, personality-less, idle, moronic bastard, can't you help me here?'

I said, 'It's not self-help I'm really looking for, thanks. I'm just trying to see if you have any books on it. Couldn't you look TS up on your stock computer and see if you do have anything on it somewhere, self-help or otherwise? I'd be very grateful.'

He said, 'It's self-help you want, mate. If it's not there we don't have one.'

My head said, 'Fuck you, you no life imbecile. Do your job and help me, you fat-assed runt. I bet no one likes you; I bet you don't have a partner. No one would go near you and I bet you reek of piss. I bet your dick's as big as my little finger and I bet your mother hates you, you sexless moron.'

I said, 'Well, thanks anyway for your help then.'

My head added, 'You fucking, great big, four-eyed sloth.'

And I gave a little wave and left with a cheery smile on my face.

It all happened so quickly. I didn't *feel* antagonistic or riled in any way, nor did I give the impression that I was. It was almost as if I'd been having a very strange three-way conversation.

That was typical of so many situations that seem to cause a separate script to run simultaneously in my head. There's a kind of duality to it, and it's sometimes confusing. Most of the time the script in my head runs an innocuous course. It says things like, 'I wonder what it's like to do your job?', 'Are you married or single?', 'Hell, you're wearing clashing colours!' or 'Mother of God! You've got a deep voice for woman!' It's a harmless, but very vivid commentary that probably verges on the normal, as you probably have a similar harmless little script running yourself. It's the extremes that I have the trouble with.

Sometimes, although not very often, I do get a little vocal. It's usually in situations when I really do think that I'm being treated badly in some way, times when most other people wouldn't react and would just stay quiet. I guess that in some tenuous way this relates to the very vocal aspects of Tourette's – not that speaking my mind is in any way a tic or even a variation on the Potty Mouth Tourette's theme. Take one of those famous American coffee shop chains, the ones where you have to queue up to be served your latte, cappuccino, espresso or whatever. The service can be awfully slow in these. You end up standing in a huge line while the assistant goes through whether the customer wants a large, medium or small mug, whether they intend to drink in or take away, if they want skimmed milk or whole, if they're opting for a single or double shot of espresso and on and on. It's endless. All I want is a simple coffee, and everyone queues in silence like grazing, half-witted cows, while it takes five minutes to take a simple coffee order. So I stand in the queue, getting more impatient by the minute, irritated at all the options available to the customer being served, irked while they hum and haw over the decision they should have made well before ordering, and furious that the customer who, having made his or her choice, then spends another five minutes fidgeting for the money they must have known would have been required at some point in the transaction. It's all too much for me. I can't keep quiet. This happened to me recently. I stood and waited, did a slow count of ten, then another and then another until, finally, I had to say something. 'I could have grown the coffee bean, milked the cow and glazed the bloody mug in the time it's taken you to serve one customer,' I said. Everyone stared at me as though I was a complete psychopath. And then those in the queue started giggling and agreeing with me. I wasn't going out of my way to upset anyone, in fact, I delivered my speech in the nicest possible tone, but I managed to get my point across. This sort of thing happens frequently now and I sometimes wonder if I'm becoming a complete vindictive busybody or if I just like to get people scuttling about. I think it's the latter, though, because when people are all of a scuttle, I see them becoming busy – their bodies becoming busy – and in a sadistic kind of way I get a kick out of it. It's nice to provoke the busying of other bodies. It makes me feel not quite so alone, I suppose.

A really infuriating aspect of my Tourette's has to do with people speaking and me listening. I very often feel as though I'm either hearing people twice, or that they are stammering. This is a hard one explain. When someone speaks, *as* they are speaking, I think that I already know what it is that they are getting to. By the time they've ended their sentence, I already know how it's going to end. I'm certainly not psychic, but I suppose I am a bit impatient by nature. I'm not just cleverly guessing what people are about to say. I presume to some point I am instinctively *feeling* what they are about to say. But whatever it is, I get really rattled when people tell me things, explain things or chat in long phrases, because I'm dying to give my response, yet they are still only halfway through what it is I'm already ready to respond to. I do know that having Tourette's – having much of the world speed into my focus and not having the ability to filter things out – makes me very impatient. But when I'm listening to people, it's like that feeling we all get when someone who has a stammer can't get the word out. That feeling of 'yes, yes . . . yes' when they are stuck on a word, that feeling of '. . . just *say* it', that impatience that makes you want to say the word for them. That's how I sometimes feel when people talk normally to me. I want to finish their sentences for them, to hurry them along and to stop them dilly-dallying over an explanation. I'm really not sure how this clinically ties in with Tourette's, but I'm certain that as my Tourette's has worsened, this stammering thing, this knowing what others want to say, has become more and more acute. I can tell you that it not only causes me much irritation, but also the talker, as he or she ends up feeling hectored, and that's never my intention. Obviously I still have some work to do with this brain conflict of mine.

CHAPTER 12

ONE LAST WORD

The wonderful feelings of happiness and safety that I was experiencing in the RCM Junior Department were to last only another year. I was in the Upper Sixth form at school and, while everyone one was going through university entrance procedures, I had to prepare myself for my audition to study full-time at RCM. My school days were happily scarce, and I was able to devote all my time to playing the piano and listening to records. I was a young man obsessed – I was on a mission. My emotional state was probably better than it had ever been and, as the days passed, I felt as though I was shedding a huge load from my back as I moved towards actually being in the wonderful musical environment of the Royal College five days a week.

The audition was successful and my place at the RCM was secured. I'd never been in any doubt that it would be the case. It wasn't arrogance; I was just in love with music and knew that the RCM was the place that would nurture me. One thing bothered me, though. The Junior Department had been intimate, with a small number of students, but the senior college had so many students. I wondered if the senior students would be as friendly, if I would I fit in there or go back to being ashamed and embarrassed because of my 'nerves', or whatever the hell it was that I had. I hadn't 'grown out' of anything; I was seventeen and still had all of the violent bodily symptoms that I have exhaustively described. I thought myself incredibly ugly. I knew I'd be meeting new people and wondered if they would make me feel worse about myself than I already felt. I feared that their normality might again prove to me just how different I was. I didn't feel ready for more tastes of harsh reality.

I wondered if senior RCM would be full of couples, boys and girls, that sort of thing. I doubted I would ever get a girl-friend when I was so ugly and stuck with my busy body. What if, what if, what if? Questions nagged at me day and night, and I became obsessed with them. I worked myself into quite a frenzy. I was so worried that I spoke to my mother about it all. I told her that I didn't think that I had the strength to actually go to RCM full-time, I told her how ashamed I felt and how I knew I had no experience of real life. I didn't think I had the energy to spend my whole life stifling tics and trying constantly to pass my odd vocal sounds off as singing practice, or something equally believable. I just didn't think I had it in me. I told her how I stifled my tics like mad each Saturday at junior RCM and that I had lots of friends. But by going full-time, they were bound to eventually latch on to my abnormalities. What if they saw the real me, the so blatantly different, freaky me? What then?

My mother must have been disturbed by my near hysteria; after all, she knew that it had always been my dream to go full-time at RCM. Suddenly I was telling her that I didn't think I could go through with it. Of course, she had no idea what torture and punishment I'd been through at school and how my fears were based on experience. She remained very calm while I opened my heart to her and listened patiently. She said she knew I'd find the strength to do what was right for me and would support my decision, whatever it was.

I guess my mother's words calmed me somewhat, and I spent the next few months literally floating through life, doing everything on automatic, not actually thinking too hard. It was my way of reaching a decision, a way of not thinking about painful 'what if's and a way of enjoying the happiness that I wanted with all my heart to continue. It was my way of keeping things as they were.

Home life, thankfully, still allowed me the luxury of being alone and undisturbed as I immersed myself, ever more deeply, into music. I was thirsty for knowledge and lapped up the great classics, the modern masters, symphonic music, chamber music, choral works and piano works. I was addicted to Bach at the time, and the works of that God among composers rejuvenated me, inspired me and, above all, helped free me from my still utterly exhausting tics, movements and noises.

Venturing from the safety of my music room into the body of our house, with its long hallways and multiple levels, got even stranger. My mother had stopped her involvement in politics and was now completely occupied with her friends and with yoga. She had taken to practising her poses in different rooms around the house, claiming that she wanted to experience all the different energies of our home. I would often open the door to our lounge and be assaulted by a strong waft of incense and find Mother, sitting in the middle of the floor in a leotard, with one leg wrapped around her neck. Or I'd go into the study to look for a book and find her in there wearing a kaftan thing, theatrically poised against the wall doing her 'tree' pose. I could do nothing but laugh, in fact, I used to laugh so hard I thought I'd pass out, and that would get Mother at it then, and she too would start giggling at the situation, eventually losing her pose entirely and collapsing on the floor in hysterics. I don't think my mother took herself that seriously, despite being obsessed with her figure. She always laughed with me at herself and in retrospect I often wonder if it wasn't all just designed to help me have some fun. On the other hand, it might have all just been sheer quirkiness. She was known, and still is, for her colourful behaviour, like the time when I was seven and she turned up to see me in a school play wearing an outrageous purple turban on her head with real fruit pinned to it, grapes, cherries and maybe even a peach.

We still had our little collection of emotionally damaged people constantly knocking at the door, but there were enough rooms in the house for me to be able to avoid them completely if I so chose, which I usually did.

Susanna was now permanently living away from home and, although she visited frequently, usually with some gorgeous boyfriend in tow, we never managed to build any kind of relationship. There was an ocean between us, and years of resentment and a lack of empathy had rendered her a stranger to me. I no longer even wanted to be her friend and it probably showed.

A particular period, in which 'ghosts' from Jeremy's old life kept visiting us, made me very uneasy. During his life he'd had two girlfriends, both of whom adored him beyond words. His was a strange life, because when I say he had two girlfriends, I mean that he dated, or rather was in a relationship with, both simultaneously, for many years. It was an odd threesome, I suppose. Anyway, these two girls started visiting us. They were both, three years on, still completely broken by Jeremy's suicide. I liked the two of them immensely, but they were opening up a very deep family wound, which naturally upset us all. I was particularly freaked out when, on one of their visits, one of the girls said how much I looked like Jeremy, and how proud he would have been if he'd been alive to hear me play the piano as I did. It was too much for me to handle. I went to my room and sobbed. I beat my pillow. I was sad and furious – sad for the lost life and the waste, and angry that the pain was still killing us all.

Tics, noises, movements, touching and all, I decided that I would brave the real Royal College the following September. I was learning that life was about moving forward and dealing with blows if and when they came. I decided that since I'd managed to get through school then anything was possible. I was starting to believe in myself, I suppose, not just as a musician, but as a person. I was learning to cope with being me in your world.

One last word on my school life will close the doors on that monstrous and destructive epoch of my life once and for all. On the last day of my very last term, just as I was about to leave the school building, I bumped into the teacher who had rolled about in laughter with the class at my expense. She was a rather masculine woman, with a particularly sour face that looked as though she was eternally sucking on a slice of lemon. She stood in my path and, looking down her nose at me, said, 'So, Nicholas, what is it *you'll* be doing next year?' I looked at her and remembered that day. I saw her laughter and I watched her encouraging affirmations to my classmates to break me. I looked at her and realised that neither she, nor any other teacher, had any idea that I had won my place at the Royal College. I knew that to her I was still a freak. A thing. A *nothing*. I understood that she hadn't asked her question out of curiosity, but out of sheer spite. She wanted me to say that I didn't have anything planned, or that I'd been rejected by universities, or that I was going on the dole, or that I was going to sit in a cage in the zoo, where, no doubt, she thought I belonged. I looked at her and all my years of torment flashed before my eyes.

And I remembered.

Unlike in class, when I'd had no answer to her question, I now had a reply. The words flowed slowly and evenly from my tongue.

'Mind your own fucking business, you evil piece of shit.'

I walked on and never looked back.

Chapter 13

Transition

God, I felt free.

School was something from the past. The days of torment were, I hoped, over forever. Nothing was going to stop me now. For the first time in my so-far jumbled and painful life, I relished the long summer holiday and didn't spend it in dread of another school year.

To top it all, I had been asked to participate in a music summer school. It was a course run by two very renowned and, as it turned out, generous and warm-hearted women musicians – a pianist and a cellist. Their summer course was for talented young musicians who wanted to learn the art of, and to explore, piano chamber music – trios, quartets and the like. Nine days in the country surrounded by music and other gifted musicians sounded like bliss to me.

I prepared for that summer school meticulously in two ways. First, I learnt the music I was required to play and lapped it up in my usual greedy musical fashion. Second, and of equal importance to me, I practised stifling my tics. I didn't want to run the risk of being judged as a weirdo by the other musicians on the course. I wanted – no, I needed – them to be able to look beyond my blatant tics and things, to see around the random and odd violence of my body's own little dance, and see the real me.

I was already used to being around other musicians my age from all those joyful Saturdays spent at the RCM Junior Department. I knew that my peers there saw beyond my 'nerves'. In fact, I managed to stifle my oddities to such an extent that most people there probably hadn't noticed that I had any. One day a week, stifling with all my might had been exhausting, but seemed relatively easy compared with the idea of having to keep up my stifling act for nine whole days and nights. So you can see why I was worried.

I tried to think of ways of disguising my tics and tried all manner of tricks to camouflage the obvious busyness of my body. Attention from rolling my eyes hard in their sockets might be distracted if I tried closing my eyes when a roll came on. Perhaps, but wouldn't that just make me look more odd, or just different odd? I didn't know and my care-fully set-up mirror for my disguise practice didn't help at all, as my eyes had to be closed during the tic, so I never got to see how I actually looked. How about coughing each time I had a verbal tic then? Plausible perhaps, but, then again, maybe not. It sounded too much like an elephant trumpet-ing. And damn, once I'd started this new trumpet thing, it too became a verbal tic, almost as if my vindictive little Touretty tic-selection panel, deep in my brain, decided that to have me trumpeting away would be rather fun.

Touching things didn't bother me too much, or rather the idea of other summer course participants seeing me touching things. I was a pianist, so I supposed that particularly quirky tic could always somehow be blamed on pianist's eccentricity. The head-shaking and nodding thing was a tricky one, though. I tried adopting a horrified or at least mildly startled expression each time I shook my head, thinking that I could pretend to feign irritation over a too tight collar, or an attack by a mosquito or something equally irksome. That sort of looked OK when I checked the result in the mirror, but was it too much? Did it just make me look more jumpy and nervous than the original tic? I didn't know. Now the nodding. Well, with that, I decided a smile would be a good idea, not that I would ever have dreamt of inflicting a radiant, full-on, 'say cheese' smile on anyone. I felt far too ugly for that. I obsessed daily on my godforsaken, dreadful looks. But I thought a little friendly look and a tight mini smile when I nodded almost looked OK. I worked quite hard on that one actually, and of all my Touretty disguises I think it was the one that came off best, although I couldn't help thinking that my smiles and nods, despite my most laudable of intentions, rendered me a cross between Bette Davis as the nanny from hell and our dear, majestic Queen at her most smugly, well, majestic. Oh well, at least I tried. Very hard in fact.

On the way to the summer school an odd thing happened. Well, not so much odd as curious, I suppose. I had to take a train from Paddington and, as it turned out, it was a particularly full train. I walked up and down its length several times before spotting a seat. Two guys of about my age were sitting opposite me. From their accents they were clearly Scottish, and as they were chatting I heard the odd word that made my ears prick up. Piano. Violin. Beethoven. Harmony. After about half an hour I could no longer contain myself. I leant across our dividing table and blurted out, 'Are you both musicians? I am!' They looked a bit shocked actually, but soon enough I discovered that they were on their way to the same music course as I, and, furthermore, one of them was a pianist just about to begin full-time study at the Royal College. His name was Alan. Yes, *that* Alan, the victim of my Touretty touching, Alan who has so much patience and understanding of my odd personality. Alan, who I met on a train – the 2.53pm from Paddington, to be precise, and I *can* be: I was wearing a blue jacket over a lighter blue shirt, he was in a pastel mauve V-neck and cream trousers, his seat was red, mine was blue and on and on – Alan who became, and remains, my closest friend.

As it was, my tics, touching and noises were never an issue while I was at summer school. After a day or so there I stopped actively trying to make my oddities less obvious and became wrapped up in real human interaction, actually dropping my guard and for the first time in my life having fun, normal harmless tomfoolery, natural and essential immature, naughty, raucous joy. You might wonder what was so big a deal about that, but, to me, it was a huge deal. You see, I had missed out on any kind of natural interaction with my peers when I was at school. All those years when kids explore their own and each other's personalities, act imma-ture, laugh about and enjoy themselves, I had been the freak. I had been actively excluded. Now I suddenly found myself being an active participant in fun. It was new territory for me.

Those nine days were full of pleasure. The music-making was so gratifying, but the camaraderie, the being accepted, the being sought out to have fun with, was worth more than mere words could ever describe. Yes, it was naive fun. Yes, it was very 'jolly hockey sticks' kind of fun. It was nothing compared to the fun that the cyberage kids of today seem to have, nothing like it at all, but, you know what, I loved it. For me it was all new. For me it was *outrageous.* I was suddenly living. I was so happy I could have cried. If I could have made time stand still and kept myself in that place, at that time, with those people, doing the things we were, I know beyond a shadow of a doubt that I would have done so.

Unfortunately, real life is never so simple.

A few remarkable events occurred at the summer school. One was rather lovely: a girl, a cellist, came up to me and asked me how on earth I could keep up such a high level of enthusiasm all the time.

'What do you mean?' I asked.

'Well, whenever I look at you, I see you giving encouraging nods to everyone, almost as if you are willing us all on, making us strive as you do,' she replied.

I mentally shouted a great big 'YES!' My nodding camouflage smile thing *had* worked, after all. In fact, it had bloody well triumphed. Never had such words been so spontaneously offered to me. The sentence still ranks as one of my all-time gems, as it was perhaps the nicest thing anyone had ever said to me. I could have kissed the girl. In fact, I did kiss her – I kissed her on the cheek and hugged the now-rather-startled creature with all my strength.

The other odd episode, which is now very amusing on retrospect, was when Alan and I had been persuaded by a kind, hearty girl to escort her to the indoor swimming pool. It was located far from the school's main building in a creepy corner of the grounds, and I think the girl felt a bit too spooked to venture there alone. I didn't fancy a swim, and nor did Alan, so we chatted by the water's edge while the girl was in the changing rooms putting on her swimsuit, or so we assumed. Anyway, all of a sudden, the changing-room door opened and the girl popped out completely naked. Alan and I nearly fell into the pool. 'Come on, you two,' she shouted, as she bombed into the water, 'Don't be shy.' I looked at Alan and could say nothing, because at that particular minute, my tics, bodily and vocal, decided to go haywire. Alan pulled a tart little face at her naked body. 'Ach, how disgraceful, how utterly obscene,' he said, in his thick Glaswegian drawl. 'Sex should only be part of marriage.' I was suddenly all of a nod, nodding not only in agreement, but also because of Tourette's. *Sex? Who the hell said anything about sex?* My head was spinning. I didn't know anything about sex. I didn't *want* to know anything about sex. Yuck, yuck, yucky, yuck. Bloody hell!

My first few terms at the RCM full-time passed pleasantly enough. I had a routine going that I loved, and I'd venture out each morning with the proverbial spring in my step, not praying that I wouldn't be bullied, not dreading what was to come, not with a feeling of nausea at the prospect of being victimised, tormented or even just ignored. In that sense, I was in heaven. As it happened, I didn't bother trying to hide my tics and things after all. It's all very well trying to plan careful tic disguises, but the real thing isn't quite so easy. Yes, of course I stifled the odd few, particularly the violent shockers, but on the whole I found myself so busy that I didn't have the chance to step back and say to myself, 'Hang on, here comes a tic. Guards up, disguises at the ready . . .'

My tics, and all my Touretty manifestations, just went on as usual. I had a great circle of friends, some new and some old, from my junior college days, and they were all odd bods in their own ways. I suppose they all just saw me as a fellow odd bod. No one ever mentioned my oddities and, in retrospect, I wonder why they didn't. Maybe they were all so kind and polite that they would never have dreamed of mentioning my behaviour. Or maybe they just accepted oddness and put it down to eccentricity. Whatever the case, they saw way beyond the noises, the blinking, the nodding, the head-shaking, the eye-rolling and the knee-jerking, and witnessed what was then developing into the real me, a me who felt safe and more confident, a me who didn't expect insult and abuse at every turn, a me who felt comfortable enough to let the real me emerge from behind the exterior me. As for being in an environment bursting with music five days a week, well, it was earth-shattering.

Since I already lived in London in a large house, and with two grand pianos, I didn't have to move away from home during my college years, as so many of my fellow students did. I was happy that way and felt I had the best of both worlds. I could spend my days at college and then go home at the end of the day and practise peacefully without having to book college practice rooms or squabble over who got the better piano to work on. The big thing of independence, having fun, 'living', severing the apron strings, all fell on deaf ears in my case. My home seemed much more interesting to me than some student bar with cheap lager and oversexed singles. My parents were so pleased that I seemed so happy with college that we were all in a constant state of delight. Worry – for they no doubt worried themselves silly over me being traumatised by my tics – was soon abated when they saw how happy and settled I was at college.

My mother noticed how settled my tics seemed. She said she even thought my 'nerves' might be leaving me. Well, that was pushing it somewhat. Of course they seemed less to her because I was out for most of the day and nowhere near her constantly watchful and tic-monitoring little eye. And I was happier than I had been in years. Happier than ever, probably. My mother was not focusing on my tics because I was growing into a confident young man, and that, for any mother, has to be gratifying. But the tics were there. The obsessions still ate at me, the compulsions to do things like spit in eyes and finger greasy noses were still compelling.

Actually, during that first year at college, I thought my tics were becoming *more* sadistic. I got worried. My nodding was more aggressive in execution, and my eye-rolling was giving me really tender eyeballs. I had a strange and persistent headache and was not in a good state at all. I decided I'd make an appointment to see a doctor local to the RCM. It had been nine years since I seen the hospital neurologist. Nine years since I'd been labelled 'attention-seeking'. I suddenly felt brave and desperate enough to give a medical professional my trust all over again.

So I went along to see this new doctor and explained that I had 'bad nerves', which I thought might be St Vitus' dance. I told her about my life, my new life, and I described my pain and discomfort. She took some notes and asked me to go behind a screen and remove my clothing so she could give me a physical examination, which I thought somewhat strange. I hadn't removed *all* my clothing for any of the other doctors I had seen. Anyway, when I was naked she came in and pressed and poked me, listened to my heart and lungs and examined my eyes. She was silent throughout. Suddenly she left the little cubicle, which I saw as an indication that the examination was over. I started to get dressed, but her voice told me to stay put, she hadn't finished. I didn't know what she thought she might achieve by examining me further. My bad nerves – or whatever they were, because I didn't know – didn't emanate from *on* my body but from somewhere *in* it, probably my brain, or so I suspected. The good doctor then reappeared in a sight that would have graced the most grisly of horror movies. She had on a thick plastic tunic, was holding up a rubber-gloved hand and was smearing lubricating jelly onto her index finger.

'WWWhat are you doing?' I managed to stammer.

'I'm going to give you a rectal examination,' she said.

Oh.

'Oh,' I said, 'but why?'

'Well, I need to have a poke around and see if anything's up there,' she replied firmly, as she came towards me, finger extended.

What the hell . . . ?

Poke around?

See if anything's up there?

Jesus!

Visions of hideous alien things lurking in the depths of my bowels sprang to mind. Images of being host to some deformed, ticcing and gyrating monster flashed before my eyes.

I'm sorry, but there was just no way on earth I was going to let this doctor person 'poke around' inside me. *No way, José!* I quickly grabbed my clothes and held them tightly around me like a little shield. 'Sorry,' I said, 'but I don't think that's really necessary. I don't believe my headaches and nerve troubles evolve from my bottom. I'm not having the exam,' I added, while eyeing her ominous and now well-lubed finger. 'Sorry.'

And that was that. No miracle diagnosis for me, and no help or cure either. To close the book on *that* little story, I must add that I mentioned my rather harrowing doctor's visit to some of my friends and two of them, as it turned out, had had similar experiences with the same doctor – the finger, I mean. One had even gone so far as to go through with the ordeal. Another friend, a girl, said, 'At least you don't have ovaries. She squeezed mine.' *Squeezed her ovaries? Bloody hell!* The doctor clearly had quite a reputation for her digital probing. Evidently the finger–orifice recipe was a technique she employed for all number of problems.

I managed to control the physical pain I was in with strong painkillers that I stole from my mother's stash of pills. Not that they really took the pain away, there was no way they really could have, as I, or my brain, was constantly making me aggravate my pain by the constant tics and nods and eye-rolling and on and on.

My mother had a huge stockpile of prescription medications. How she managed to procure them all I really cannot say to this day. She certainly didn't take most of them herself, but held them as a miracle panacea for other people's ills. She was constantly palming out pills to all and sundry. 'I've got such a headache,' one of her friends would say and, in a flash, Mother presented them with an opiate painkiller. 'I'm so stressed,' another friend would say and, hey presto, there was Mother offering a tranquilliser. It was all so, well, clinical, for want of a better expression. If you had a symptom, then Mother had the cure. From flu remedies to tranquillisers, all the way to anti-psychotic medicines, Mother had it all and so convincing was she in her assurances that 'one of her little pills', as she called them, would do the trick, that people happily accepted them and even claimed delightedly, often only seconds after taking one, that they were indeed cured. It was amazing. It was also paradoxical; none of Mother's magical pills had any effect on my 'bad nerves' whatsoever.

I never quite realised then just how eccentric or alternative my family actually were, but, in retrospect, they were loopy in the extreme.

The house was large enough for my parents to live almost entirely separate lives, and this set-up suited them both rather nicely, because they rarely saw eye to eye.

While my mother did her yoga, handed out pills and paid court to the never-ending flow of bleeding hearts that passed through our door, my father became more insular and self-contained by the day. He's a bit of an enigma, my father. In his younger days he had been a judo champion and captain of the British and European teams. He'd lived in Japan for a number of years to study judo and spoke Japanese fluently. In fact, he had come fourth in the World Judo Championships in the days when there were no weight categories separating contenders and he'd been beaten eventually only by a giant of a man. When I was very young, say three or four, I have memories of a very bold and confident man, always dressed sharply in the best of hand-tailored suits, dangling a massive cigar from his mouth. Now, he was introverted and unconventional.

He retired from his job the year I left school and decided to do the thing he'd always dreamed of doing. No, it wasn't a world cruise or an exotic golfing holiday for my father. He grew a ponytail. It was his little statement of nonconformity and it rather suited him in a funny sort of way. He'd also taken to sculpting heads, not out of clay or granite, but out of apples. It was quite creepy actually. Every few days or so we'd find a head sculpted from an apple sitting proudly on the dining room table. Invariably the head would be a kind of caricature of someone in the family – one time me, then my mother, sometimes Susanna and, other times, it would be a self-caricature. They would sit there, these weird little heads, turning browner by the day and shrivelling so all the features became distorted, until they had shrunken beyond all possible recognition, when they would be replaced by a new one sculpted from a fresh apple. My father also played the flute, and his own obsessive nature used to see him tooting away like a crazed blackbird trying to perfect pieces of music. I suppose that, given the choice, he would have chosen some kind of artistic career, but his family's social situation never allowed him to follow such a path. Instead of this making him bitter and discouraging of my artistic ventures, he encouraged me in my pursuit of excellence and made sure he was able to provide an environment in which I could thrive.

Susanna had moved to Japan to teach English and was, by all accounts, having a whale of a time, although I suspected she was running away from her own demons related to family life and Jeremy's suicide. I was long past the point of holding any kind of grudge because she hadn't been able to relate to me as a 'nervy' boy; I now felt the absence of a sister who I wanted to finally get to know.

The house was a busy little world in itself. It was wonderful that I could escape its bizarre inhabitants, well two of the three, and shut myself off in my music room where I could play the piano at any time of the day or night, and furthermore, where I could tic as hard as I needed to in absolute privacy.

In my college life I started having a few problems. After the initial thrill of actually attending a high-powered music college, I realised I wasn't getting on well with my piano teacher. Incompatibility between teacher and pupil is nothing rare in music colleges, where the relationship is on an intensive one-to-one level. I guess not every teacher is suited to every student, and I just wasn't finding my lessons as inspiring or instructive as I'd hoped. I didn't feel I was learning enough and, to make matters worse, a member of staff had begun nodding at me, in imitation of my affliction. As a result, my tics seemed to worsen again, as did my general emotional state.

On paper I was doing well. I had played some acclaimed concerts and had even been awarded an exhibition – an award for excellence for which first year students had to compete. But something was missing.

Instead of living for music, I clung to my friends, to Alan in particular, for he was the most understanding person I knew. Alan had his own teething problems with the RCM. He was living away from home for the first time in the college halls of residence and he hated it. He was also unhappy with the way things were panning out at the RCM and, like me, seemed rather disappointed with the whole set-up. I suppose we supported each other through that year as we both found our feet and dealt with our traumas. Even though my tics became rather outrageous and Alan couldn't but notice, he never said anything about them. He neither commented nor judged, and I appreciated that. He just *knew*, and his knowing made me feel not quite so alone.

Midway through the year, I made friends with a girl who was a very talented harpist. We bonded and became inseparable. We would spend hours listening to music together, playing music together, admiring each other's musical gift and encouraging each other – something I certainly needed as I felt nothing of the kind was being given from the RCM. She was bold in her attitude towards music, curiously masculine, and I was enthralled to find another person who was so ambitious, so alive and so driven by music. She too never commented on my tics, but funnily enough her best friend did. The friend, an adorable Irish girl, was a violinist and we were by chance in the same class for musical history lectures. Anyway, once she got to know me she was bold enough to say what it turned out she had been busting to say to me from the first term: 'I looked at you in class, and I thought to myself, "Oh, that poor, poor boy, with those dreadful tics."'

That was it. I wasn't in the least bit offended. She was a warm and genuine girl, and there had been no malice behind her words. I didn't tell her about my nerves or the suspected St Vitus' dance. I said nothing. I didn't want to explain anything to anyone. I wouldn't have known where to begin.

Towards the end of the first year, relations with my piano teacher reached an all-time low and, in truth, I felt I was not learning the things I needed to equip me as a pianist.

Regrettably, the situation was becoming unworkable, and I was at a loss as to how to deal with the unexpectedness of it.

I jointly won the end-of-year piano prize for first year students. Six of us had been nominated to compete. I remember that I hadn't been particularly inspired when I performed, but clicked onto automatic and went through the motions, letting my touchy Touretty fingers do what they did best. I hadn't worked on the pieces passionately or in great detail with my teacher, and winning seemed not to make a great deal of difference to the way I felt about my lessons. There was bad feeling from some people in the college because I had won, and, what with feeling no enthusiasm from my teacher, I began to dread the idea of another three years of the RCM. I began ticcing badly again. The old stomach-punching thing reared its ugly head again and I was finding it hard to keep up with end-of-year high spirits.

At home, we decided to get a lodger. With so many rooms and so few people, my parents opted to rent a room to an English language student who would get to experience English family life, such a batty example of it as ours was. Our student was a middle-aged Japanese woman, who spoke not a word of English, had pots of money and delighted in drinking heavily and offering all manner of drinks to anyone who happened to be around. She was an absolute darling and I grew to adore her. She evidently liked us all enough too, as what was meant to be a stay of three months ended up being three years. I once went into our dining room to find her sitting in a chair, cocktail in hand, toasting our dog, who, himself, had been poured a good dose of whatever it was that she was drinking. She was very dippy, and she fitted in rather nicely.

Despite not even having a basic command of English, our Japanese student saw that I was in a hell of a state. I can't imagine what she thought I had. Come to think of it, I didn't know what I had either, so she wasn't alone. She insisted on massaging my tight and painful neck and shoulders, pressing all kinds of secret little pressure points on my body, in order to relieve, or try to relieve, me of my symptoms. She never did manage to stop my busy little body in its movements, but at least she managed to give me some mental calm, which at the time made all the difference.

My now close friend, the harpist, finally mentioned my tics. 'I don't know what you've got,' she said, 'but you're going to end up in hospital if you carry on like this.' I was at my worst. My vocal tics were especially bad – I was yelping and blowing raspberries for England. My head-shaking and nodding had hurt my neck so badly that most of the time I had to hold my head up with my hand, because my whole neck was so tender and weakened. I was so very tired.

'Come with me to my parents' place in Wales for the summer,' she suggested. 'You can escape there. You can rest. You *need* to rest.'

God, how I needed to escape and rest. I wanted peace and, if it so happened that peace was to be found in Wales, then Wales was where I would go.

Chapter 14

I'll Show You Obsessions

Obsessions are very strange things. I'm certain that most people have, at some time in their life, experienced an obsession. But what exactly is an obsession? I'm sure most of us can remember having had a crush on someone at some point during our lives. Maybe it was the proverbial teenage crush, or possibly it happened much later in life. That feeling of desire, that 'I must have' or even 'I'll die if I don't have' is a very powerful thought indeed. You think of the person all the time, you imagine what they are doing; in fact, the object of your desires consumes you. But is this urgent desire so very different to an obsession? I don't believe it is, not when we talk about such a burning desire. It's not like me wanting a cappuccino, or desiring one. It's not like you dreaming of buying a new car or fancying a great wedge of chocolate fudge cake. Those desires, presumably, do not consume us during each waking moment, and if they do, then we probably need some type of professional help. So what *do* people become obsessed about? Well, some people seem to be rather obsessed with television, especially soap operas. (Or is that simply an addiction?) Some of us are obsessed with our appearances, liking to be pristine all day, every day. (Or is that just vanity?) Many men and women are obsessed with tidiness; overly house-proud people who smugly make others feel that they live in filthy flea-pits. (Or is that just being neurotic?) Some people are indeed obsessed with a constant desire to eat naughty things, those secret bingers who stuff sugary, fatty things down their gullets when they think no one is looking. (Are they just plain greedy?) Well, the list could go on and on.

So what really does constitute an obsession? I think that any continuous or repetitive thought or desire that actually interferes with quality of life, or has the power to directly command certain aspects of life, is a true obsession. People throw the term obsession around so much that the true meaning has been all but completely obscured. Of course, there will be periods in your life when you think of a particular thing or person a heck of a lot, but it's not really a driving obsession.

This wonderful expression, Obsessive compulsive disorder, or OCD, seems to have become very popular of late and is generally thrown casually around much like 'anally retentive' is, or 'I'm depressed, I need Prozac.' Medical professionals must be in heaven now, because all of a sudden, as if it had been an airborne virus launched from outer space, everyone and their dog appears to have OCD. If someone likes washing their hands a lot, they have OCD. If a child won't work at school, but only wants to play, then he has OCD. Someone depressed from being laid off from work . . . must be OCD. The teenager who can't seem to stop phoning chat lines and running up her parent's phone bill . . . of course, OCD.

There is no end to it, and I hear people dropping OCD in all the time when they are chatting. I hear husbands complaining about wives who have OCD. I hear teachers talking about pupils who have OCD. I hear mothers talking to their friends about their toddlers, and telling them, as little Johnny takes out his willy in the middle of a coffee shop, that yes, he's got OCD.

Either there is some perverse conspiracy with the aim of trying to convince everyone that they have OCD, or the term is quite clearly being misused.

Even Tourettists, families of Tourettists and help groups for TS, throw the term OCD around very casually. I'm certain that they also use it far too frequently, or even erroneously. Obsessions, rituals and compulsions very often feature in Tourette's, and it is wrong, I think, to extract them, label them OCD and see them as something in *addition* to Tourette's. A Tourettist's desires and needs to do or think certain things stem from Tourette's itself. TS is home to many characteristics and features under its large umbrella, and obsessions are in there. Someone who is told that they or their child has TS *with* OCD is being misled, for it's probably just the case that the TS is more profound in that person. A person who has obsessions *and* Tourette's has the OCD as a *part* of the TS, not as something separate. I am, of course, aware that many conditions are genuine examples of OCD and totally separate from Tourette's syndrome, but that, in itself, should really deter the term from being thrown about so casually.

As a Tourettist, I'm consumed by a huge number of real obsessions, some of which are what I'd call minor ones, while others must definitely be considered major because they are absolutely implicit to my overall well-being.

It's strange that over the years, my obsessions have changed and adapted themselves to somehow 'tune in' to the various stages of my life as I've grown older. The things I obsessed about when I was eight were different from those at eleven, sixteen, twenty and now. I can't say that I have more mature or important obsessions now than the earlier ones, because the thing about obsessions is that whenever they occur, at whatever age, whether they are about toys and building blocks, or rocket science and everything in-between, they are always valid and equally important.

I have severe obsessions *because* I have Tourette's syndrome. That is a fact. But this obsessive aspect of TS doesn't just confine itself to good old-fashioned and simple obsession. Other obsessive aspects also occur, sort of mutant obsessions, which I know stem from exactly the same little compartment in my brain as the TS gene. Things like ritualistic behaviour, self-mutilation and destructive thoughts.

Tics, motorised movements, the desire to spit in left eyes, touching things and abusing people in my head are not compulsions or rituals. They are things that I do not think about but just happen, anytime, anywhere.

I suppose that my obsessions, and all the things associated with them, grew and became part of me in synchronicity with all the explosive or violent bodily Tourettisms. There was no time when I suddenly just discovered that I was obsessing or behaving ritualistically, no sudden realisation at all. It all just crept up on me, and gradually began to consume me mentally, just as the bodily tics were doing physically.

I actually obsess over far more things than I could ever jot down in this book – things like constantly tweaking my computer settings until my PC just gives up and dies. That's a horrendously consuming obsession for me. I lace and unlace my shoelaces again and again, threading and unthreading. I ritualistically line my shoes up pointing towards the door each night before I sleep. I'm obsessed by house plants – I hate them. I feel they are sucking in the air that I need, and, like in *Day of the Triffids*, conspiring against me. I know it's another completely wacky Tourettism, but I can't help it. I get really freaked out when I go into someone's home and see all manner of potted plant things staring at me defiantly. Of course, I know they're not really out to get me, but I can't *not* obsess that somehow they might be. I obsess about having to have wax-free ears and am always poking around in them with a cotton bud. I ritualistically have to pee, or squeeze pee out, once an hour every hour, sometimes even on the hour. I also ritualistically close every door twice, whether I'm entering, leaving or even opening wardrobe doors. I obsess over my forehead, where there is a wonderful little point that I press hard, for hours on end. It gives me a wonderful sense of peace, as well as an unfortunately large bump, which, of course, I know is utterly ludicrous.

Another ridiculous ritualistic obsession – one that's almost scary – happens whenever I'm standing on a platform waiting for a tube train. As the train approaches, I'm obsessed with the idea of jumping into its path and, in fact, often move so suddenly and swiftly to the edge of the platform that people get startled, probably thinking I really am going to jump. This is not suicidal behaviour, but more of a pest of an obsession, a 'what would happen if' kind of thing. It's almost as potentially dangerous as something that happens to me when driving on motorways. I'll be moving at speed and will have to close my eyes for a slow count of ten while releasing my hands from the steering wheel. Luckily, despite my brain telling me to keep my eyes closed, I always peep while counting, so it's not as potentially lethal as it sounds. As with the tube train, this ritualistic obsession is more in my head (like most obsessions), than in good old reality.

I also obsess over music, which could be considered natural because I am a pianist, after all. But I've spoken to many, many pianists about this, and none have ever given the slightest hint that they obsess over music in the same way I do. Not one waking moment goes by when music is not consuming me, where my fingers are not motionlessly playing a piece of music, or when my brain is not visualising notes on a page, or, most of all, when I'm not hearing musical works in my head. I don't mean that I'm silently humming the tune of something, or that I'm practising a particular piece silently or even that I'm merely hearing snippets of something. I hear pieces, works, symphonies and operas loudly in my head, in the booming speakers of my brain – whole works right through from beginning to end. The music is full force and vibrates its sonority through every cell in my body. I feel it. I'm not just imagining how the piece goes, I'm living a performance of it – it never switches itself off. If the phone rings and I have to talk to someone, the music will continue, but will reduce itself, rather considerately, to being low-volume background music, until I finish the phone call and am able to have it back full blast. It never pauses, and never stops. In fact, I often don't even make the selection of what I'm going to hear. I feel as though I'm a walking iPod, with no 'off' button. This isn't the same as a run-of-the-mill 'think' obsession, where the recipe consists of thinking about the same things over and over, it's almost an independent obsession that just goes on endlessly in my head, consuming my thoughts, all by itself.

Some of my obsessions are not as pleasing as the music, though. Some are painfully destructive and downright scary. Take my nail-biting. Lots of completely normal people bite their nails, not just nervous ones, as we are often led to believe. My nail-biting is destructive and obsessive. It's destructive because I'm a pianist and could really do without biting my nails down to the quick, and it's obsessive because I don't just nibble them but have to practically rip them from my fingers every few days or so. I dig my teeth into the nail, or rather I dig an incisor into it, I get hold of a bit, bite and then rip as much away from my finger as possible. It's agonising, and rather like some awful Chinese torture, where I'm both the torturer and victim at the same time. I do this with each nail, often drawing blood along the way, and, if I'm unable to actually bite off the right amount, which varies, I'll grasp for anything sharp – a knife or scissors usually – and dig it in until I'm able to *peel* a satisfactory and satisfying amount of nail away. This nail-biting is not a tic in any way. It's more of an obsessive ritual, and one which happens to be rather common among Tourettists. It's blatant self-mutilation. I cannot control this, and nothing will make the desire, the *need*, go away.

My longest-running and most potent obsessions are to do with my physical appearance, my looks. These aren't somehow a case of self-worship, or just plain vanity; quite the contrary actually. I used to hate the way I looked, and this self-hate is one of the constants that, as an obsession, is still with me today. As a child I was consumed with being ugly, buck-toothed and puffy-eyed. It was how I saw myself, and is what I reminded myself I was, day after day. In my twenties I saw an ugly young man whenever I looked in the mirror. The self-hate was like an anchor around my neck at a time when looks seemed to be so important. People would see me examining myself in the mirror, and assume I was being out-rageously vain, when in truth, I was just assessing how flawed I was. Today I'm still obsessed with that same feeling of ugli-ness, of being riddled with imperfection.

It would be very easy to think that all the self-loathing was due to me having been teased so badly at school – called freaky and ugly. But it all started long before the teasing began. It's a *major* obsession, one that will not leave me and one that nags at me every single day. But here's the odd bit. While I'm consumed with thoughts of ugliness, while I obsess over my 'flaws', I know that in reality I'm not ugly at all. It's all very odd. What stares back at me when I look in the mirror actually bears no relation at all to what my obses-sive thoughts tell me I'm seeing.

My obsessions are part of me. I suppose that somewhere along the line they helped to mould my personality. They don't ruin and haven't ruined my life and they don't make me an unbearable person. They are just another feature of my busy life as a Tourettist.

CHAPTER 15

PANDEMONIUM

The following academic year at the Royal College began, and I soon launched back into life as a music student. I was refreshed after the long and lazy summer that I'd spent at my friend's house in Wales, where I'd been able to be myself in all my ticcy glory, with no risk of comment, judgement or even sympathy.

I ploughed straight into music and began my seemingly never-ending practice routine all over again. I was still troubled by an absence of inspiration and, still having the same piano teacher, I lacked enthusiasm for my lessons. In fact, there was a huge distance growing between me and my teacher and it was rapidly becoming a stalemate situation.

Towards the end of the first term, the RCM paid host to a world-renowned pianist who had spent all of her life in the USSR and never been allowed to travel abroad. Now that barriers were down and the political climate had eased, she was allowed out for the first time, and one of her first ports of call was to be the RCM, where she would play a recital and conduct a masterclass, which is a kind of lesson, an imparting of wisdom, a judgement even, given in public to an audience. Tatiana Nikolayeva was her name, this monument of Russian piano playing, and six RCM students were selected to play to her, myself being one of them. Furthermore, while the other five had chosen to play bog-standard Chopin, Brahms and Bach, I had selected a massive piano piece by the Russian composer Dmitri Shostakovich, a work that it just so happened had been composed for, championed by and premiered by Nikolayeva. I was laying myself open to a potential slating, Russian style, and visions of Nikolayeva standing over me and shouting 'Nyet, Nyet, Nyet' started to haunt me. In preparing for the masterclass, which promised to be attended by all number of musical bigwigs, I was pretty much left to my own devices. I'd played the piece to my teacher a handful of times, but with our working relations being what they were, I had to rely on my own instinct to get me through. I had to understand the music I was playing, had to be able to play it technically perfectly (it was fiendish), had to ensure that it was safely in my memory and, most of all, I had to make sure I could convey its meaning and project it to an audience. I couldn't help but feel that I was on my own.

My tics and things were rather considerate to me while I was battling away to learn my piece properly. In any case, I was giving what they wanted the most – concentration. In fact, I barely gave them the chance to surface.

The day of the masterclass arrived and I felt as though I'd either throw up from nerves, or else have an accident in my pants, although I preferred the idea of the former, given the choice. First off was Nikolayeva's recital. She was a small woman, about as wide as she was tall. She seemed ancient, and kind of resembled everyone's idea of a Russian peasant washerwoman. But when she started to play the piano it was nothing short of magical, which made me all the more terrified at the prospect of playing to her.

The masterclass began, and instead of listening to the first few students, I ran off to get my head in order, to find the strength to go up there and play myself. Alan kept running back and forth to the opera theatre, where the class was being held, and giving me updates. 'She's ripping them to shreds,' he said, wickedly, and I just thought, 'Oh God, she's going to eat me alive.'

My turn came. There was a large audience, and I was suddenly up there, on stage, with Nikolayeva sitting a just few feet from me, next to her translator. She asked me to play the whole work through. I did. For the first time in my life I think that I played magnificently and the applause when I finished was rapturous, but the question was, did Nikolayeva like it? That was all that mattered. She eased into her opinion by sharing some of her experiences with me, with the audience. She spoke of how she'd been presented with the piece by Shostakovich, how she'd worked with him on it, how it had been the culmination of everything he'd wanted to say in piano writing. Then she stood, beckoned me to stand, and came to me and kissed me on both cheeks and embraced me in what felt like a bear hug. She was so warm and cuddly, but she had this enormous mole thing on her chin, with a prominent whisker projecting from it, which tickled my chin as she kissed me, and I hate to say this, but everything else faded into oblivion and I was overcome by an urge to touch her mole, or tweak the hair, although I didn't. Anyway, of my playing, she had no criticism, and said that I was already a pianist. Then she congratulated and hugged me again. There was more applause and suddenly it was all over.

A few people who were not directly connected with the RCM came up to me and congratulated me. The founder of the Leeds International Piano Competition pumped my hand furiously. The actress Shirley MacLaine, who had come to watch the class because she was starring in a film about a guru piano teacher called Madame Sousatzka, kissed me, and even my piano professor gave a pert 'well done' as he passed by. From the rest of the RCM, however, only one member of staff and three students congratulated me. I was unaware of any encouraging noises from anyone else, and it felt as though there was a great college wall of silence, although I had no idea what it was that I might have done wrong.

I decided to change piano professor and study with another member of the RCM piano faculty, a man who enjoyed quite a reputation as a pianist. It just so happened that he had been the only actual member of the college's staff who had congratulated me after the masterclass, but that's not what made me choose him. It was instinct, and one that proved to be spot on.

With my new teacher a whole world was opened for me, one of colour, sonority, textures, refinement, elegance and, above all, conviction. I had lessons three or four times a week, often for many hours at a time. He made me aware of things I never knew existed in music, things that I had never dreamed were possible with the piano. I won another RCM competition, then another and then another.

However, I still felt as though the RCM hierarchy remained silent. I was disappointed and felt more than a little hard done by and unappreciated; they seemed blind to my successes, deaf to my talent and immune to my passion.

I tried to find out what was holding me back at the college and questioned a few of the professors that I got on with. They told me that I didn't fit the college mould and that some people mistook my passion and dedication for arrogance. *You can't fit a square peg into a round slot. You play with too much passion. You can't relax into college life. You run at full throttle and that seems to upset the powers that be.* It was very revealing actually.

My old piano professor once told my mother on the phone that I was the 'Arthur Scargill' of the RCM, so obviously I did come across as a militant. I guess I was right in everyone's face and that made me seem pushy. I also think I may have come across as overly ambitious, and although that shouldn't be a cardinal sin in itself, it can certainly alienate one. But, in truth, though, I wasn't bitingly ambitious: I was just so desperately and ruthlessly driven from inside – from the Touretty me. There was no ambition for ambition's sake, but simply an adoration of music – an obsession with music being the purpose of my existence. In retrospect, I'll admit that my manner at the RCM might have come across as somewhat arrogant, perhaps because my experiences at school had left me fearful of becoming a victim again. But I never felt I was being arrogant to anyone there. I believe I was just running on a kind of overdrive that I was unable to control. I think it's a shame that the RCM didn't feel inclined to accommodate someone who was quite clearly different and in trouble. Perhaps I expected more from the college than they were able to give, or maybe it's just that they expected something different from me. I never got to understand.

I didn't change my ways. I couldn't. My approach was somehow wrong for the RCM and I couldn't somehow fit into one of their peculiarly shaped slots. And that was all there was to it.

In my third year I went to see the director. I was devastated by yet another knock-back and I wanted to know what all the negativity, what all the nastiness, was about.

'You are undoubtedly one of the finest talents the college has ever had,' he said. 'But you must realise that many of our members of staff once aspired to be what you are now aspiring to and it's possible that some of them don't like to see in you a passion and talent that was maybe lacking in them.'

Bloody hell.

I was almost speechless and I was all of a quiver, because I'd spotted the director's bony knee – it was staring right at me – and my fingers started tingling, and I was dying to give the knee a bloody good, ten-fingered squeeze. My brain was screaming orders at me to touch the knee, but I was there to deal with much more important things.

'So where does that leave me?' I asked, while eyeing the knee.

'Well,' he said, 'if you don't like it here, you can always consider leaving.'

Are you kidding?

Thanks.

Thanks for nothing.

And that was that. It really was. I didn't leave, but I sure as hell spent as little time as possible in the college building from then on. I still carried on lessons with my professor, though, and still loved learning with him, but as far as college was concerned, it was over.

One interesting, yet still musical, experience helped act as an antidote to all the problems I was having at college. My piano professor, who had worked as the musical advisor on the film *Madame Sousatzka*, was asked to help another actor who was preparing to play the part of the composer-pianist Frédéric Chopin in a film (which was later called *Impromptu*). The actor's name was Hugh Grant, and it was to be my professor's job to try and make him successfully mime at the piano and make it look as though he was actually playing. Well, I was at my professor's home when Hugh first came by for a 'lesson', and it was fascinating to watch as he, having no keyboard dexterity at all, was taught to mime to a recording. As things turned out, my professor discovered that he was not going to be able to spend as much time with Hugh as he would have liked, so he suggested that I take over the tutoring. I was thrilled.

Hugh Grant, who was not quite the household name he is today, came to my house everyday for a week to intensively learn how to mime, move and generally look as though he was playing the piano. He was extremely friendly and receptive and, furthermore, seemed to be exactly the same in real life as he always is on the big screen. It was also amusing, because, in order to realistically portray Chopin, who was consumptive, Hugh was on a crash diet consisting solely of grape juice, in order to gain the washed-out, sickly look necessary for the part. The poor guy was famished and sat grasping a pint glass filled with grape juice, swigging furiously whenever he could.

It was during my college years that two hugely significant issues came to light. Both related to the whole future course of my life and both were realisations of the fundamental me.

Growing up, going off to music college, homing in on my ambitions, all in all doing what I wanted *and* doing it in a safe environment, led me to start thinking about girls. A girlfriend was the next step, if I went on what I saw most people of my age doing. My father asked me if I'd met any interesting girls at college yet. I watched other guys lusting after girls when I went to the pub with friends after college. But there was one major problem: girls just didn't do anything for me. Other guys seems much more appealing.

I suppose I've been gay, or known that I was gay, for as long as I can remember, but during my adolescent years, when boys are supposed to have an erection three hundred times a minute, when they are supposed to be dreaming of sticky gropings, I really didn't give sex, or my sexuality, so much as a thought. It wasn't that I was in denial; it was simply because I had been driven by things, which, to me, seemed so much more potent than sexuality. I had been engulfed in two worlds, one of music and the other of Tourette's. Both are greedy. While other boys of my age were no doubt immersing themselves in sexual fantasy and wet dreams, I was dreaming of performing, of being a great pianist, of getting through the next day at school unharmed, of waking up one morning to discover to my delight that I was cured of all that made me so ugly and freaky. In any case, I knew from family and friends how much worth is given to physical looks in the gay world, and I knew that I was ugly. I obsessed over my ugliness. I never thought I'd stand a chance in the gay pecking order, never even be in the running. So you see the whole gay thing had never been in the forefront of my brain or my emotional needs. There was no great big queen sitting impatiently inside of me just bursting to jump out.

I decided to take the bull by the horns and 'come out' – tell my family and friends I was gay. I never felt the need, as do so many gays, to scream, 'I'm queer and I'm here!' or 'Come to me, sisters!' or 'Here I come girls, ready or not!' I'd met loads of gays over the years though my parents. I'd seen gays of all shapes and sizes at the RCM. There was just no big deal.

It all happened rather suddenly, the coming out thing, and it all happened because I decided that I'd start wearing contact lenses instead of glasses. I know it sounds shallow, but it was not until I saw myself *without* my great big tinted goggle things that I decided, despite the evil little Touretty 'whisperings' to the contrary, that I was actually quite OK-looking. That's how it happened. I looked in the mirror, thought 'not bad at all' and went downstairs and told my mother what was what. Mother poured herself a large gin and said she was so happy that I wasn't a drug addict or something nasty like that and that she had no problems whatever about having a gay son. 'Here's to the queers,' she said as she toasted me. Jeremy had swung both ways anyway, she told me. Now that *was* news to me.

My father was a different ball game. I left it to my mother to tell him, and I remember playing the piano furiously while she broke the news.

'Your mother tells me that you *think* that you might be a homosexual,' he came in and said to me.

'No, Dad,' I said. 'I *know* I'm a homosexual.'

He was really upset for about a week. He cried and said that he was mourning the continuance of the family name, mourning the grandchildren he would never have from me, scared that I'd lead an ostracised and lonely life.

I could say nothing to convince him otherwise, so inconsolable was he. But then, wearing dark glasses to hide his puffy eyes, he went off to see a friend of his who was gay and when he came back he was a new man. I don't know what passed between the two of them, but I can honestly say that my father has never once uttered a single word of negativity in relation to my sexuality. He accepted it and moved forward, and I admire the way he handled it. Actually, at one stage he was so curious to know what the gay scene was all about that his friend took my father to a gay evening run by a gay support group. There, my father chatted with all number of elderly gays and some, to his delight, were dressed in drag, while others were genuine transvestites – a big, burly truck driver with a moustache, dressed in a flowery Laura Ashley dress actually asked him to dance. My mind boggled.

Susanna was still living in Japan at this time, and my mother relayed the news to her on the phone. Susanna and I had had no real contact for a very long time, but apparently she had a mixed reaction to suddenly discovering she had a gay brother. On the one hand, she felt admiration for my courage in coming out, and, on the other hand, she felt guilt. You see, she went through an initial thought that I'd been permanently put off women because she'd always been so nasty to me, and because of the way she and her friends had acted around me. Then she startled my mother by admitting that she thought she might have emotionally scarred me by something she'd done to me when I'd been just a baby. Apparently, when no one had been looking, she'd undone my nappy and twisted my little willy round and round tightly like a corkscrew. Mercifully I have no memory of that.

So, gay I was, and I told Alan as much when I next saw him. As my best friend, he had to know. I did a long build-up and then dropped the bombshell, expecting horror, but Alan just shrugged and said, 'Ach, well, you know, I'm exactly the same way.' We rolled about laughing, especially when I reminded him of his tart little look and comment about sex being disgusting and only part of marriage, one he'd made when we'd been green and innocent. Now, it wasn't a question of Alan and I falling into each other's arms and living happily ever after. Not all gays are like that, you know. No, we were friends, and friends are what we've always remained, through thick and through thin.

Alan and I had endless fun exploring the gay scene together. We started out as scared little boys, petrified when some lecherous old queen pinched our bums, and we ended up years later rejecting the whole scene thing and just getting on with our lives. It was something we had to do, a process we had to be part of.

The curious thing about all those years of harmless fun, getting to know other gay men, flirting, cruising and all that, is that I never felt secure within myself. Oh, I could get to know people, I could always end up with any man I wanted to be with, but I never relaxed. It was the Tourette's. I was never able to let go for fear that someone might have seen the real me, the ticcing me, the noise-making me, the hyperventilating me. People used to be attracted to me physically, but were invariably 'put off' for want of a better expression, when they actually spoke to me, when they got the wrong vibes from me, when they realised that I was very closed as a person, not forthcoming, tense and intense. It was all due to my huge complex. The huge complex that said, 'Whatever you do, don't let them see you tic, don't let them see what you are, don't let them in on your ugliness.' The inner conflict I had that was constantly waging war in my head was staggeringly destructive. On the one hand, I felt good-looking and sexy. I thought I was probably desirable. But I was flawed and I knew I was because I was constantly being told I was from deep inside. Despite the fact that I could sometimes disguise my obvious tics, despite the mirror giving me a nice reflection back when I looked into it, I still heard those jeering voices from years ago saying, 'You ugly bastard, you ugly fucking freak.' I was petrified that people I met, those with whom I flirted, would realise that I was damaged – with tics, noises, thoughts, complexes, obsessions and desires. Things that would either open me up to humiliation, or else subject me to ridicule. So I let people see the surface me, but that's all they got. Nothing more. I could neither let them get emotionally or physically close. It was just too much of a risk for me. Of course I wanted to give more, to successfully flirt and get to know people, but I simply didn't dare, at least not until I trusted them.

I suppose that sexually I'd been very naive as a teenager because I was so wrapped up with the constant fight of trying to tame my own body and its wild and uncontrollable movements. I'd spent no energy on any possible sexual urges, mainly because I had no energy available to give. So as a recently 'out' gay man with more sexual awareness than I'd ever had and so much temptation before my eyes, my engines were on and I was raring to go. But unfortunately, the gay scene was like a meat rack. If you didn't fall into your role as wild sex stud within the first few moments of meeting someone, no one had the patience to explore further when there were so many other available and much easier pick-ings. So, while everyone else seemed to be getting on with the job and having wonderfully exciting little flings and flingettes, I remained alone, the person who flirted wildly all night, but went home alone.

My lack of success in the 'partnering' game set a pattern that I was unable to break for many years. That's not to say that Alan and I didn't have a whale of a time. We were exploring and growing up. It was all new. We looked at the world, the gay world, our gay world, through our thankfully naive eyes and forever lived in hope and dreamt of the leg-endary Mr Right. We shopped together, chose outfits, screamed when we had a big red spot, got to know other cool gays, learned to avoid bitter gays, got drunk and mastered the art of cruising. They were somehow magical days, and they provided stark contrast to the stilted and negative atmosphere we associated with the Royal College. But I never managed to conquer the almost demonic fight that was going on in my head, probably because I had no idea what the fight was, why it was there and if it was normal. I guessed that everyone had their own little demons. I just had no notion that mine were unconquerable.

CHAPTER 16

A REVELATION

The other thing that happened that would have such an impact on my whole existence was much more earth-shattering than coming to terms with being gay. I finally found out what I had, what the demons were that had been affecting me for so many years. I discovered that what had caused so much heartbreak and misery was, in fact, Tourette's syndrome – Gilles de la Tourette syndrome, to be precise.

My tics and noises, and all the usual stuff that had been going on in peaks of severity for so many years, had reached another all-time low. I decided to see a doctor, but my family doctor this time. I wasn't going to be lured in to the grips of a rubber-gloved, finger-probing doctor again, no way. So I toddled along to my family doctor, the doctor who had seen me practically since I was born and had referred me to the specialist neurologist all those years ago. I told him that I couldn't cope anymore, that I was losing it, I was being consumed. I stressed that I had really, really not 'grown out of it' and that I honestly wasn't continuing an attention-craving act.

My doctor referred me to a different hospital's neurology department, where I was seen by an honest lady who said that whatever I had was way out of her area and that I needed to see a real specialist. I have to say that that lady doctor suspected Tourette's syndrome, but didn't tell me. I know this because just last week I sat down and read through my entire medical file, which is kept with my GP. But I'm jumping the gun. I was given an appointment with yet another neurologist and I went along to his clinic and was questioned and examined by a panel of doctors. Childhood memories of this type of visit came flooding back. The main doctor – the one who I later found out was the actual consultant, the specialist – said very little to me. He took me through my symptoms, history and the rest (*he* didn't suggest any digital probing), and that was it. It was over.

'I'll write to your GP,' he said as he dismissed me.

I didn't quite know what to make of it all. I suppose I should have asked 'What do I have?' but I was so stunned by his rather uncommunicative manner that I didn't think to.

I went back to my family doctor a week later, and he showed me the letter that had been sent to him. It said that I have Gilles de la Tourette syndrome. I looked blankly at the page. It said nothing to me.

'What's that?' I asked my doctor.

'I haven't got the foggiest idea,' he replied. 'But the consultant does say how we might treat it. Meanwhile, I'll find out what it is.'

It was almost funny, but it really wasn't.

I had a syndrome. I had a real condition. They knew what was wrong with me. I had the classic symptoms of Tourette's syndrome.

Questions raced through my brain. *What the fuck? I've had it all these years, this real syndrome? It obviously affects other people? There is some treatment? I have the classic symptoms? How could the doctor have known what I had, when no one else had spotted it? Why did no one tell me I had it before?* Questions, on and on.

I was furious. I was so angry that I could have screamed. In the next few weeks that anger became more profound and with their new-found name my newly christened Touretty things got worse and worse. I was angry and Touretting wildly.

I did some research on Tourette's syndrome. For God's sake, I found that there were associations for Tourette people all over the world – help, support groups, advice and channels of contact with other sufferers. My research confirmed that I did indeed have TS. There was no doubt. I'd been seen by countless neurologists when the symptoms developed all those years ago. I'd had close encounters with rubber-gloved doctors and I'd endured humiliations, agony, tears, family devastation and utter desperation. Fourteen years later, I was being told that I did have a real condition after all, and not just some godforsaken, absolutely unknown, attention-seeking madness. *'Bad nerves', stress, 'nervous tics', 'attention-craving', Valium, 'ignore him', 'he'll grow out of it', homeopathy, child guidance, bullying, painkillers, confusion. Nooooooooooooooo!*

I felt that the medical profession had failed me. Completely. Something that distressed me greatly was that TS has been in the ambit of neurological information since 1885. Every doctor whom I'd seen had obviously been totally unaware of it, despite my demonstrating the most obvious, textbook symptoms of the syndrome. I'd been treated with Valium, which, as I later discovered, has never had the reputation of being able to deal effectively with any tic disorder, TS or otherwise. That information was apparently documented in the 1970s when I'd first been prescribed the drug. And surely any keyed-up doctor should have realised that they were dealing with something a little more unusual than simple old 'bad nerves', even if they had no notion that such a thing as TS existed. I'm certain that the doctors I saw did not get such vivid and violent examples of multiple tic syndrome every day, so, being as one might hope at least clinically *interested* in their patients, why did no doctor ever think to explore or do some research? I'm sure if they'd looked, Tourette's syndrome would have screamed from the pages of some medical textbook somewhere. The years of humiliation and anguish that I endured might have been slightly lessened had we had a legitimate name for my condition. I might not have felt quite so alone and it would have been heartening to my parents to know that we were not the only family experiencing such worry.

I was also angry because, having waited for fourteen years to find out what I had, the doctor who finally and correctly diagnosed me hadn't even had the courtesy to tell me what was wrong with me. I'd had to read it in a letter he sent to my GP. He surely could have said something along the lines of, 'I'm sure you're *dying* to know what you've got,' or '*I* know what you have,' or come straight out with: 'You've got Gilles de la Tourette syndrome. Shall I tell you about it and our research?' But I got nothing. I felt like a specimen, maybe another statistic in some neurological research. Obviously I didn't deserve to be personally told what I had.

So there I was, twenty-one, and I knew what I had. I tried the pills that had been suggested as a treatment, but they had absolutely no effect on me at all, which is quite surprising really, because when I looked up what they were, they turned out to be a powerful anti-psychotic drug, one that is usually used to treat lunacy (charming!) or other violent conditions. It seems that there had been some success with the drug in Tourettists, when given in small doses, but with me, even though I increased it to see if I would benefit, there was still no effect.

I stopped taking the pill and had to endure a long wait until my follow-up hospital appointment. It was during this time that I started being able to piece various things together. I found out as much as I could about TS. The World Wide Web was not the powerhouse of information we all take for granted now, so I had to leaf through obscure books in libraries. I even made contact with some other Tourettists and was able to quiz them about their own experiences. It was fascinating and in between college, socialising with Alan and my piano practice, I would delve and delve, constantly learning and always trying to understand. A few interesting opinions on Tourette's popped up. I read some odd articles that suggested that TS was more likely to occur in people who originated from hot climates; my mother is from South Africa, so that got me thinking. I read accounts of people who had been burnt alive in the Catholic Inquisition for being possessed by demons when, in reality, they were simply suffering from TS. I read that full frontal lobotomies had been tried on people who suffered TS symptoms, just to shut them up and calm them down. I found that electric shock therapy had been used. Straightjackets. Gags.

Extractions of the tongue in medieval times. I read about the tics, the yelping, the noises, the self-inflicting of pain (like my stomach-punching and nail-biting), the spitting and the obsessions. I even saw some articles that said that TS sufferers can err towards substance abuse, have suicidal thoughts and sometimes even kill themselves. So what about Jeremy then? He'd had tics. He'd been jumpy. He'd certainly suffered obsessions. He'd been a heroin user *and* he'd committed suicide. Had he also had TS? Somewhere along the line, could I link Tourette's, and all that goes with it, to Jeremy's death? I thought of my grandmother and her supposed St Vitus' dance, and the torturous hot and cold baths. It was obvious that she's had Tourette's too. There were so many questions, and while some clearly had answers, others remained in rather murky and certainly untested waters.

I tried another drug that was thought to have some effect on Touretty tics. It was a potent anti-psychotic drug called Haloperidol. It worked. It calmed me and stopped my head racing, stopped the real world whizzing through my consciousness and almost stopped all of the tic activity. But it took away my personality and it extinguished all that was me, all the personality that made me who I was. Basically it turned me into a bit of a zombie. I no longer had any spark for life or will to do anything. I'd lost my zip, become a cabbage, and would have probably remained one had it not been for my parents and Alan. They'd watched my personality literally slipping away before their eyes and decided that enough was enough. No sooner was I off the pill than I started to live again. My tics came back full-force. My head raced. I was back to being the busy body that I am, but at least I felt alive.

CHAPTER 17

A PECULIAR SYNDROME

I think that by now you certainly have a pretty good idea of how Tourette's syndrome affects me. But since in my account I've only just been told that I have Tourette's, I thought I'd pause here for a moment, and put this very peculiar syndrome in its historical and medical context. My research for this book primarily comes from me, and, in that sense, I play the dual role of being both researcher and research material. But for the more technically-minded or curious, or anyone who still doubts that such a syndrome as I've been describing could possibly exist, I thought it might be an idea to give you some 'proper' data, but not too much of it.

> *Tourette Syndrome is a medical condition with a genetic component but is as yet of unknown cause. It is characterised by a combination of chronic muscular tics (twitch-like movements) and vocal tics (involuntary noises) and is often socially stigmatising.*

Tourette Syndrome (UK) Association

In 1885, Georges Albert Edouard Brutus Gilles de la Tourette (1857–1904) catalogued descriptions of nine patients who were suffering from multiple tic disorders. One of these ticcing specimens was the Marquise de Dampierre, a well-known noblewoman, who had first come to the attention of another French physician in 1821. Apparently she suffered from both severe tics and also the uttering of obscenities. On studying the histories and symptoms of these individuals, Gilles de la Tourette was able to ascertain that they were all suffering from the same condition. The syndrome now bears his name, although thankfully in a slightly shortened form.

The symptoms of the syndrome, which apparently usually appear before the age of eighteen, usually around seven, contain an endless possible variety of tics, which on the whole tend to limit themselves to the upper body, but in the most severe cases of Tourette's, or the full-blown syndrome, can occur in any part of it. Vocal tics are usually added to this recipe and then come the possibles – the obscenity uttering (coprolalia), repeating words, echoing what has been heard (echolalia) and touching. The symptoms of Tourette's vary from individual to individual, and it seems that the syndrome makes each person almost personalise their own particular Touretty repertoire.

There are also the so-called associated disorders, like OCD – the obsessions thing – and Attention Deficit Disorder (ADD) in children, although, from my own experience, as I said before, I really don't think these are *associated* disorders at all, but mere *parts* of Tourette's. Just because a person can have these 'associated' disorders entirely independently of Tourette's doesn't render them associated if the person happens to have TS. I believe that when they occur in a person who has clear TS then they are *part* of the TS, not just associated with it. But there's no medical proof, and many professionals would undoubtedly disagree with me, but then these professionals rarely have TS, so who knows best, the Tourettist or the non-Tourettist?

Anyway, since its discovery in the nineteenth century, it is interesting that, although there has been considerable research, the most frequent conclusion seems to be that nobody knows exactly what TS really is.

Oh, they know for sure what the symptoms *are*, but the 'what's and 'why's remain the mystery. The general view is that TS is likely due to abnormalities in various regions of the brain, including, possibly, the frontal lobes (at the front and probably where our personality lies), the basal ganglia (a collection of nuclei deep down in the white mushy stuff of our brain) and the cortex (where our information is processed). These abnormalities could be caused by the way information is passed between the various regions of our brain by neurotransmitters, which pass around the data. Basically, I suppose all that means is that there are communication problems in the brain, although I'm sure it can't possibly be as simple as that.

One thing researchers seem sure of is that TS is hereditary and that Tourettists stand a fifty-fifty chance of passing the gene on to their children. Gender also seems to play a part in it, and males who inherit the gene are three to four times more likely to develop the syndrome than girls.

There is no cure for Tourette's, just a plethora of medicines that have been noted to have a beneficial effect on some Tourettists. It's trial and error really, and I suppose that it's impossible to find a cure for something if you don't know what that something really is. It must be like looking for a needle in the proverbial haystack. There are ongoing studies, though, ones that try known medications on the symptoms to see if they help. Some even seem to think that nicotine helps, but that's not just to get Tourettists smoking. The problem with so many of the medications that seem to help Tourette's is that they often provoke very unpleasant side effects. Some seem to all but eliminate the personality, others leave the Tourettist confused and sleepy and some can even cause an irreversible condition called tardive dyskinesia, which is a continuous tremor, usually of the mouth and tongue, or the fingers. It is often ironic that, in gaining possible relief from tics, TS sufferers may run the risk of acquiring something equally, if not more, disturbing.

It does seem that the very physical aspects of TS are usually totally misunderstood, often by the people who have the syndrome, their families, colleagues, parents, teachers and so on. Even family doctors seem to have trouble believing that the tics and things are entirely involuntary.

On the other hand, TS is clearly being misdiagnosed now that it seems to enjoying more widespread publicity. I often hear of people who have been diagnosed as having TS and when I'm told about their symptoms, which are often nothing like TS at all, I really start wondering what our neurologists and doctors think they are doing. I was recently asked by a friend to meet the worried father of a fifteen-year-old boy who had been diagnosed as suffering from TS. He had been seen by several specialists because of unruly behaviour at school, excessive rudeness and headaches. After quizzing the father about his son I knew that there was no way on earth that the boy was a Tourettist. He displayed no Touretty symptoms. None. I told the father this, and advised him not to let the doctors medicate his son for TS, as had been suggested. I recently heard that the boy is fine now and has got over whatever it was that was affecting him. This just isn't right. Just because a child swears in class or cheeks a teacher, it does not make them a Tourettist. Just as it is criminal that so many doctors miss quite blatant examples of TS in their patients, it is equally criminal, I think, that it is being dished out as a diagnosis willy-nilly. It's a complex syndrome for sure, but with such obvious symptoms, is it really so hard to accurately spot? I think not. Of course people can have a milder form of TS than I do, but the trademark signs will always be there somewhere.

What is heartening is that Tourettists are often known to have certain rather pleasing personality traits. Dr Oliver Sacks, the author of *The Man Who Mistook His Wife For A Hat* – a book that examines several odd neurological disorders, including TS – said in an interview in 2002: 'I think people with Tourette's syndrome often have unusual wit and velocity of thought and brilliance of association.' He also said, 'Tourette's is not all fun, it can really tear one apart and make life very, very difficult. But it can gift one as well, which makes it sort of complex.'

So there really are two sides to every coin.

While some Tourettists suffer from learning disabilities, many sufferers lead normal lives. Some even excel in their professions – surgeons, pilots, musicians, sportspeople – so it's not always something that renders people incapable. I believe that TS often *allows* people to excel, because of the way it seems to crave concentration, which in turn provides relief to the sufferer by calming the symptoms.

Over the past few years research has also suggested that TS affects far more people than was previously estimated. It was initially thought that TS affects one in every 200,000 people, but now opinion seems to be that it's more like 1 in every 1,000 boys and 2,500 girls. I even read somewhere recently that some neurologists believe it affects, although very mildly, about one in every twenty people. The jury still seems to be out on that one, but what is clear, though, what people must start to accept, is that TS is not as rare as it was once thought to be.

Unfortunately, despite the frequent references to it in the media, the syndrome remains relatively undiscussed. I really feel for all the thousands, probably millions, of people who are suffering with their TS but don't know that TS is what they've got. I know there's no cure or effective treatment, but at least having a name for your condition makes you feel less alone. I know, because I've been there. TS research and TS awareness still has a long way to go.

Finally, it must be appreciated that TS occurs in all countries, in every culture, in every race on the planet. It is not specific to any one region or people. If you start looking, I bet you'll start noticing Tourettists all over the place.

CHAPTER 18

THE TEMPLE

It was a strange feeling. There I was, trained to the highest level, equipped and experienced enough to give concerts, bursting to perform, full of music, hopes and passion, and what did I have? What was in the pipeline? Nothing. A big, fat, empty zero.

The music profession seems to work by a code I never managed to crack. Could I get an agent? No, only if I already had concerts booked. Could I get concerts? No, only if I had an agent to book them. Could I get a piano-teaching job? No, I needed references from a previous employer. How could I get references? Only by being employed. No one had told me all that during the years I was at music college. I'm sure the local education authority, who happily paid all my fees, had no idea how badly their money had been spent or how poor my job prospects were. The only possibility of earning any kind of living seemed to be to get some private students. Private piano students are the strangest of creatures, or rather their parents are, because sadly, the bulk of the private teaching market focuses on children. Oh, Mummy and Daddy will happily pay their lawyer massive fees for pushing paper, cheerfully pay their dentist half a month's wages for a few crowns, but will they fork out big bucks on piano lessons? Of course not. They want the cheapest deal they can get, and just because it's a nice little hobby for little Joey, they assume it's a hobby for the teacher too and pale if you mention a half-hourly fee that dares to reach double figures. And to top it all, the poor teacher usually has to listen to Mummy saying how talented, how *Mozartian*, little Joey is, when the reality is that he's tone-deaf and would much rather be watching MTV than practising his scales. Oh, I knew the realities of private teaching only too well. I had done it many times. In fact, I'd had a nice little practice going once. But I can't keep my mouth shut. Whether from a perverse kind of Touretty directness or just out of plain honesty, I would tell parents who waxed on about their little darling's keyboard agility exactly what I thought. I just couldn't smile, take their measly fee and think of England. Come to think of it, if they'd been paying me double or triple the fee I still couldn't have done it. I suppose I was my own worst enemy.

I was also not prepared to prostitute myself around or creep up to the 'right' people, just to get concerts or teaching work. It would be misleading if I told you that the music world isn't full of people who make empty promises, people who really could help but don't or those who are threatened by direct, in-your-face talent. It's swarming with them.

I tried to ingratiate myself with agents, critics and music-school heads, but found most to be so patronising and full of bull that I soon gave up on the whole idea. I remember one of the critics for a national newspaper telling me that all manner of opportunities would materialise if I let him have his 'wicked way' with me. 'Legs open, doors open,' he said lecherously. 'Get lost, you filthy old queen,' was my response, and I suppose word got about that I wasn't one to give into piggy charm. So I was left with nothing. I was not going to creep and crawl for measly crumbs. No way.

I had an appointment to see my Tourette's consultant. My tics were getting too much again and I hoped that maybe there had been some wonderful new medical break-through, the birth of a fabulous anti-tic, anti-Tourette's pill or something. But there hadn't. There was still no such thing. My consultant decided to try me on a pill that he said might at least help my state of mind, which in turn could help the tics and things. Might. Could. It wasn't another character-zapping anti-psychotic medicine, but a new-generation anti-depressant drug called Seroxat, which was apparently helping Tourettists to some degree. Well, I was willing to give it a try, and, after a few weeks on it, I actually started to feel better within myself, and better about my full-time role as a Tourettist. Maybe the anti-depressant aspect of it made me feel good, not that I was clinically depressed before starting it. It wasn't that I suddenly felt gung-ho great and energetic. I'd been that for years, or had tried to be. It was deeper than that. I suppose that on that secret little level where we all feel our doubts, insecurities and fears, I began to feel less doubtful, less insecure and less scared. I felt good. So my Touretty mental health was in top form, but what about the tics? I know for a fact that my tics won't just subside if I feel great, just as they won't necessarily explode when I'm feeling down. But on Seroxat, they curiously did subside considerably. Or maybe it wasn't so much that they subsided, but more that I wasn't so bothered by them. But that wasn't all. People around me – my parents, Alan, other friends – noticed a huge improvement. Of course I still ticced, but the excessive violence of the tics and all their unruly little friends had clearly abated. And, for the first time in ages I started seeing myself as not bad looking at all when I looked in the mirror, rather than just plain ugly. That was a major breakthrough in itself.

The new feeling of well-being that was given to me courtesy of a pill rendered me somehow more perceptive than I had been before. I felt too good about things to hassle myself with music-profession networking, and, on the odd occasion that I did happen to meet an agent, critic or educator who might have helped me had I crawled, I ignored their empty promises and made no attempt to promote myself among people who I felt only had something to offer at a price. Instead of partaking in the competitive game that all my ambitious peers were so fervently playing, I found myself observing them in their attempts to stand out from the crowd. I found the sexual approach to success particularly amusing – the girls who dressed to kill, in order to catch the eye of anyone with influence who happened to be straight, and the gays who often seemed to be willing to drop their knickers for all and sundry in the hope of getting a way in. Maybe the pills helped me see exactly what was going down in the world of classical music. They certainly gave me the strength to realise that I didn't want to be a part of it.

The Seroxat also made me laugh a lot. I was suddenly able to laugh away things that would normally have been an issue and got me down. I became able to laugh at myself, at the unquestionably funny things that Tourette's sometimes made me do and at the helplessness of my situation. I even found myself being more gregarious and able to laugh and find humour in almost any situation, so much so that I think people who met me for the first time saw me as unserious and rather superficial. Oh yes, I certainly laughed, and if laughing had been a criminal offence, then I would have been charged many times over, and, in my naturally very laughable defence, I would probably have chortled, 'It's the Seroxat wot done it, m'lud, it's the Seroxat.'

So I went from being a rather disillusioned pianist and Tourettist to being an extremely jovial and vivacious one. But was it the real me? Well, that was the question, but I really think it was me, as I'm still like that now, many years later. So was it indeed the Seroxat wot done it? I don't know. I think the Seroxat helped me leap over what was becoming a very steep incline, probably the incline that led to an acceptance of what I really was. What I am. As my lovely family doctor said to me when I first started the Seroxat, 'It helps to clear out all the rubbish, Nick. It really does.' It did.

Through some family and friends I was offered some concerts, some in the UK and some abroad. Not great earth-shattering venues and not particularly well paid, but such was my state of mind that I did them happily and to rather a lot of acclaim. After one of these performances I was backstage chatting to a local reporter when in walked an ex fellow student of mine from the RCM. Will came backstage and warmly congratulated me on my concert and said he'd always admired my playing, but that he'd barely spoken to me in the four years we'd been students together as he'd always found me a bit 'frightening'. I couldn't believe that anyone might have been scared of me, but it just reinforced my view that I, as a Tourettist, often ended up giving out seriously wrong vibes. Will and I laughed, and began a friendship that would last many years.

I did acquire a few private students just for pocket money, but I restricted myself to teaching only adults. At least they didn't come to lessons with a pushy mother in tow very often. It was quite hard acquiring them, though, as I had to advertise, and, in order to only attract adult students, I naively and stupidly printed the words 'Adults only' in my advertisement. Numerous furiously breathy phone calls to my house ensued, with people undoubtedly imagining that I'd invented a variation on the teacher/pupil-kink theme, which somehow involved a piano. Perhaps I'd have made more money if I'd explored the possibility; maybe I'd have even carved myself a nice little niche in the flesh trade. But I opted for the cleaner route and amended my ad.

I spent a great deal of time socialising in those post-college, Seroxat years. That's not to say that I went off, or in any way neglected, music. I still lived and breathed it, still practised seven or eight hours a day and still heard it in my head constantly. But I balanced it by living a normal life, albeit one of constant laughter. It was healthy. I had finally found equilibrium.

I developed a wonderful friendship with a girl of my age. She'd studied at the Guildhall School while I'd been at the RCM and she'd been their star pianist. Amber was, and still is, beautiful and sultry, with a sharp tongue and a wonderful sense of fun. Like me, she'd spent her whole childhood locked away at the piano – the ugly duckling with glasses and pigtails, to use her words. It seems that she'd undergone that same transition to contact lenses as I had and, with it, the matching realisation that she really wasn't bad looking after all. Well, Amber and I certainly made up for any childhood fun we'd missed out on and used to rollick about probably doing what a psychoanalyst might call rediscovering the child within us. She was as deadly serious about music as I was and facing the same closed doors in the music profession. We took time off together. Like Alan and Will, Amber became a confidant, accepting my Tourette's and moving straight to looking beyond it. Through the years, Amber and I laughed and cried together, empathised, advised and grew.

An unexpected opportunity came my way. Our Japanese lodger, the one who gave cocktails to the dog, had been back in Tokyo for a few years and had set up an English school, which, despite her own rudimentary grasp of the language, seemed to be doing rather well. With my father's help, she'd recruited teachers from the UK, but suddenly found herself a man short and asked me if I'd like to go to Tokyo for six months to help out. The idea strangely appealed to me, not least because it would give me the chance of earning some decent money for once. I had adored Michiko when she'd lived with us and the fact that she'd given up the drink and decided to become rigorously Buddhist made me curious to see her.

So I said my teary goodbyes and headed off to Tokyo. Michiko seemed odd, though. She was decidedly cold when she met me at the airport, and, back at her little apartment, where I was to stay, she remained cold and distant and spent hour after hour in prayer at an odd miniature temple she'd set up in her lounge. I didn't quite get it really, but everything was new to me and I wasn't going to try and analyse why Michiko was acting like a nun with her legs crossed. It must have been the jet lag or the food, or both, but my tics went berserk within a few days of arriving in Tokyo. Michiko, who had been so helpful and kind when she'd lived with us, now looked at me as though I was the Antichrist in person when she observed my busy body at its busiest. 'Pray,' she said. 'Pray to Buddha.' Oh God, I thought, what have I let myself in for? The idea of living for six months with the now-holier-than-thou Michiko started to look like a life sentence. I heard, from one of Michiko's other English teachers, that her Buddhism wasn't mainstream at all. In fact, he said, it was a cult, rather like the Moonies. He went on to explain that one of the requirements of his job was to attend 'the Temple' twice a week with Michiko. 'Jobs are hard to come by,' he said, 'I go to keep her happy and my job secure.' I looked at him dubiously, but his parting words gave me the willies: 'Be careful,' he said. 'Be *very* careful.' *Crumbs!* A shiver ran down my spine, and I started ticcing for all I was worth. I wondered what the hell he meant by 'be careful'.

Michiko eventually asked if I would go to the temple with her, and out of sheer curiosity, I agreed. I had visions of a dusty, icon-filled little shack, thick with incense. But I couldn't have been more wrong.

It was a massive, ultra-modern building of monumental proportions. People were flooding through its gates by the thousand and they all looked cool and detached, like Michiko. Inside, the temple itself was a vast auditorium. I had to kneel next to Michiko among, I guess, about 10,000 people, who all stared straight ahead in silence. They were like androids or something, and I realised that I was in the worst possible setting for a potential verbal tic attack. 'Your life is going to change,' Michiko whispered in a wavering hiss that sounded like a geriatric rattlesnake. 'Wait until you see her.' *Her? Who in God's, or maybe Buddha's, name is Her?* My knees were beginning to ache from the kneeling and I wondered what was going to happen. Suddenly, a screen from the stage was pulled back and, on cue, everyone sank into a grovelling bow – except me. Sorry, but if a show of some sort was about to start, then I was sure as hell not going to miss it. Up on stage, as far as I could make out, for I was sitting a way back, was a woman, sitting at what looked like a dressing table, brushing her hair. I couldn't suppress a giggle, but such hostile glares were fired in my direction that I figured I'd better hold my tongue lest it be surgically removed. There was chanting and moaning, people writhed around on the floor talking in tongues, and all the while 'Her' on stage carried on brushing her hair, or whatever it really was that she was doing, with her back to us, which I thought rather rude seeing as so many people had obviously turned out to see her. Then it was suddenly all over. The screen closed as abruptly as it had opened and I was left with Michiko, who looked dreamily at me and said 'See. See. See.'

'Um, no actually, I don't see. See what?' I said.

She ignored me.

When we arrived home it started. Michiko started shouting and screaming at me. 'Your way is wrong,' she yelled. 'You must learn, you must love her. You will.'

Please.

Love 'Her'?

Her with the hairbrush?

Get a fucking life.

As I shouted back, Michiko put her hands over her ears and closed her eyes. I could have slapped her. God, I lived in a bizarre enough Touretty world of my own, and now it seemed as though I'd ended up in a place of real lunacy. And I was in Japan. Alone. I went to my room and Michiko went out. Later that night I ventured to the kitchen to eat something but there was no food. None. I decided to go to bed.

Next morning, to my amazement, there was food in the fridge – home-cooked stuff – and nice jugs of green tea. I was ravenous, and stuffed as much food as I could. Michiko was nowhere to be seen. I decided to go out, but the door was locked from the outside. I was trapped. The bitch had locked me in. I tried the phone. It was dead. Shit. What to do? What was happening? I started to feel so desperately tired. My body got heavier and heavier. My eyes were closing. I just needed to sleep.

I woke up thirty hours later, feeling as though I'd been hit by a train. Michiko was standing over me. I half expected her to have tied me to the bed, and memories of Kathy Bates in *Misery* came flooding back as I frantically looked around for a sledgehammer. 'You *will* love Her,' Michiko said.

'Fuck you,' I replied, with feeling.

When she went to pray, I packed as quickly as I could and stumbled out of the front door as fast as my legs and brain would allow. I was dizzy and nauseous, and as I tripped along it felt as though I was floating.

I took a cab to the airport, and while I was waiting for an available flight to London I realised what had happened. I had been drugged. Things started adding up. The sudden arrival of food and the locked door spoke for itself. I don't know what Michiko had hoped to achieve. She'd probably laced the food with a mild hallucinogenic drug, or miracle brainwashing powder, thinking that after a 'trip' I'd think I'd seen the light and worship 'Her' with the ridiculous hair-brush thing. Michiko had been brainwashed, for sure. Why, or how, I still don't know, but the Michiko I had once loved was long gone. I really should have gone to the police, or the British Embassy, but I had visions of being disbelieved and escorted back to Michiko's place. I wanted out. I wanted to be home.

My tics played up badly in the few weeks after my Japan experience but, instead of being disturbed by them and fighting the unbeatable, I sort of glided through, not sure if I was finally learning that spending my life stifling the tics would get me nowhere, or whether I was in a heightened state of acceptance, courtesy of Seroxat.

Whatever the case, I fell back into my old routine of practising the piano by day and socialising by night.

Chapter 19

All at Sea

My friend Will had landed a cushy little job playing the piano on a luxury cruise liner. It wasn't a case of playing tinkly background music or show tunes, but a serious gig, which saw him playing two proper fifty-minute recitals a week, getting paid a fortune for doing so and living on the ship as a fully paid-up passenger with all the trimmings. I had planned on flying out to meet him at some exotic port and spending a few nights on board, but a better opportunity came my way. The cruise company evidently felt that giving their passengers a culture option worked well, and they requested a few more pianists for other ships. Will recommended me and I had to throw some musical programmes together and fly out to meet a ship in Osaka for a three-month contract. I was thrilled, although there was a certain discomfort in having to fly back to Japan so soon after my near miss with the brainwashing squad.

My three months on ship were more like a massive holiday than a job, for which I was being paid more money than

I'd ever dreamed of making. My twice-weekly concerts were not only well attended, but managed to become a highlight of the voyage for so many of the passengers. I soon got over the initially very odd feeling of performing on a slightly rocky, sometimes horrendously so, stage. Moreover, I was gaining more and more performing experience and learning to feel less fazed by the stress and nerves of public performance. I also learned the art of public speaking, something usually foreign to musicians, who are generally quite happy to play to a large audience but would wet themselves if they had to even recite the alphabet in public. I loved speaking to my audiences, bringing the music alive for them, helping them to appreciate what they were hearing and, more importantly, bridging the usually massive gulf that lies between performer and audience. I became more and more confident and enjoyed swanning around the ship's decks chatting to the audience who travelled with me, relishing their compliments and feeling like a celebrity. In that tiny world at sea I *was* a celebrity. I was someone, and I loved it. It was a far cry from the frightened and victimised teenager with enough emotional baggage to sink an oil tanker.

The cycle of ship for a few months, home for a few months was something that would last for nearly five years. I can honestly say that during that time my Tourette's was never an issue, for me or for anyone else. Yes, I still ticced and blinked and nodded and the rest, but I felt so energised and powerful that it never got me down. I mentioned before that my tics almost vanish when I perform, so the ship put me in a position where I was performing almost all of the time. I don't mean just my concerts. It was much more than that. You see, ships are rather small worlds. Each lot of passengers who boarded (the turnover was fortnightly) got to know that I was 'the classical pianist' and therefore every time I stepped out of my cabin there would be whisperings of 'There's the classical pianist' or people would say 'hi' or they'd chat to me about music or their own musical experience, or concerts they had attended, or how they were enjoying the cruise, or how they wanted a recording of me, or about my musical education. And on and on. So in reality, every time I walked out of my cabin into the main body of the ship I was 'on'. On stage. Performing. To me I was just being myself, but to the passengers, to my audience, they were chatting to one of the ship's stars. What to the other 'stars' on board was an annoyance, an invasion of their time offstage, was to me a delight because I felt that I managed to fool my Touretty brain into believing I was performing and, consequently, all my exhausting and painful Tourettisms subsided. The tables had finally turned. Instead of spending most of my day ticcing and nodding and touching, etc, all that was now reserved for my time alone in the privacy of my cabin, which was usually just a few hours at night before bed. Whatever I did, whether sunbathing on deck, dining in the restaurant or breezing around cocktail parties, was virtually Tourette-free. No one ever noticed that I had a busy body.

Living on a ship is socially rather curious. I initially thought that it would be hard to make friends among the staff of the ship – the ship's company. I had envisioned cliques and bitching and griping, but to my surprise I rarely met anyone who was remotely that way inclined. Instead of being a new boy in a world where friendships had already been sealed – for most people who work on ships usually sign long, long contracts – they welcomed new faces and accepted me easily. The diversity of the captive souls on every ship I worked on proved fresh and stimulating, and I developed many, what I can only describe as transitory, friendships. Normal friendships. No freak, no afflicted, no victim in sight.

I was in an environment where I was able to thrive, and the fear that my peers back home might turn their noses up at what I was doing didn't even enter my head. I was relieved of a massive bulk of my Tourette's, travelling the world in luxury, playing concerts, getting paid a small fortune, forming friendships and basking in the confidence that stardom, albeit on a mini, mini level, was bringing. I was even getting the odd proposal of marriage, usually from stinking-rich American widows, who would often shower me with gifts, ranging from expensive watches to a thousand dollars cash slipped under my cabin door, with their compliments. It was all very flattering.

During my months on land, I relished in my new-found confidence, from having had my ego repeatedly stroked while at sea. I also had financial security, which never lasted very long as I have a compulsion, which I believe emanates from Tourette's, to spend, spend and then spend more. But there was no problem with that, because I always knew that I would be going off to sea again where I would earn more.

After years of indifference, my relationship with Susanna was getting stronger. Almost on a whim, I decided that it was time to visit Susanna and I went to Portugal, where she had relocated, determined that we would, as more mellowed and mature adults, be able to overcome our differences once and for all. We climbed over and cleared the huge hurdle that had endured for decades and were finally able to see each other more objectively and with a new respect.

After living the glamorous life of going to meet ships in exotic locations for nearly five years, I decided that it was time to anchor myself back on dry land. Great as the cruising had been, the novelty had long worn off and I felt I was due for a change.

Strangely enough the struggle to make a living that had ensued before was not nearly so prolonged this time round. I didn't butter up all the 'right people' or drop my pants for the predatory music profession's gay mafia. I just gently asked around among my small circle of friends to see what might be available to me. My now dear friend Will proved again to be generous and helpful. It was a strange friendship really, because on the one, main, level it was just a case of two guys who were great friends, but on the other, Will was fired by ambition for *me* – he had complete respect and admiration for me as a pianist and I think he was only one of a small handful of people who believed that I should be performing, recording, teaching and touring on the international music circuit. It wasn't a love thing. Will was never in love with me or mesmerised by me. It was just that he, as he kept saying, 'saw my worth'. In any case, it was through Will – his contacts and his suggestions – that I eventually managed to get a nice little practice of good private pupils (not children), become a music examiner and do some teaching at the Royal College of Music, of all places. I also started being an adjudicator, or judge, of the numerous competitive musical festivals that are held all over the UK throughout the year. I was gradually falling into the routine of what was expected of a musician in his late twenties, and funnily enough I was quite content.

I still played and practised the piano as hard as ever, but not with the same goal. I had a handful of scattered concerts lined up, but decided not to strive or fight for more.

I enjoyed the examining and adjudicating immensely and, instead of living that bitter little music-profession cycle that sees examiners and adjudicators being as vindictive and scathing to the candidates as their own examiners and judges had been to them, I encouraged, respected and applauded candidates in their efforts. That's not to say I was overly lenient when examining instrumentalists or that I gave everyone a first prize in competitions. Nothing of the sort. But I tried to make all criticism constructive, balancing each negative with a valuable positive. I had no intention of ever making anyone feel negative, for I knew only too well how damaging that could be.

There was one major problem, though. The familiar Tourettisms had got steadily worse since I'd given up the cruising. I suppose it was inevitable that they kicked back, having been satisfied and calmed by my sea 'performing' for so long. Not that they affected my teaching, examining and adjudicating; they were happy while I was busy. But it was on the days when I wasn't professionally busy that they started to crave attention and *make* my body busy. The tics and nodding and all the rest gradually became exhausting and detrimental to the quality of my life. The cycle was repeating itself for the umpteenth time.

I was also developing an odd intolerance to the Seroxat, experiencing nausea, hot and cold sweats and particularly wild nightmares.

An appointment was made, and I trudged back to see my dry consultant. I had gradually weaned myself off the Seroxat because of the side effects, and he decided to try me on Prozac. I was quite chuffed actually. The idea of throwing in to conversation the odd, 'Of course, I'm on *Prozac* now,' rather appealed to me. It was also suggested that I have a mammoth brain scan, known as a PET (Positron Emission Tomography) Scan, for Tourette's research purposes, some educational 'tests' and an appointment with a behavioural therapist because I was back to obsessing myself into a coma for being so ugly.

Well, I didn't fancy having to vomit out my entire ugly obsession thing to an analyst, so I missed that appointment. He might have got the wrong idea about me and I didn't want to create more confusion. But the educational tests, I decided, would probably be OK. I went along to the appointment for these and sat down with an earnest lady who sat opposite me holding a pack of cards. I wasn't sure if she was a magician and about to show me a few tricks or if she was the resident soothsayer and about to tell my fortune, but as it turned out, she was neither. She arranged the cards on a table face up and told me to look at them, which I did. Nothing hard, so far. She then turned them over and asked me to find the pairs. So I did. All of them. First time. Still nothing hard. 'Oh,' she said. 'Let's try that again, but *properly* this time.' *Properly?* I didn't know what she meant. So we did it all over again, face up, then face down, then all the pairs. She took the cards from me, looked at them, held them up to the light and said, 'Let's change the pack.' *Change the pack? Did she think I was cheating or something? Did she think I had clever little X-ray eyes?*

So we repeated the whole thing over and over, and then with different cards with different symbols on them, and then different shaped cards. She then asked me to read a paragraph from a card, which she then took from me and proceeded to question me on. Instead of answering her comprehension questions, I just said the text, which she was now holding against her breast, back to her verbatim. 'Oh,' she said again. And that was pretty much it. On the way out she said, 'You're not normal, you know?' 'I know,' I said, as I waved goodbye, thinking, you don't know the half of it, honey.

The brain scan became the brain scan that never happened. Well, I went through all the pre-scan stuff, like choosing music to listen to while I was actually in the machine because I'd be in it for many hours, having a head mould made for me out of plaster of Paris, so that my head would remain still throughout. Everyone was terribly nice, but just before I was to go into the scan machine they presented me with a document, which they asked me to sign.

'Why?' I asked.

'Well, it's just to get your consent to do the scan, and to show that you've understood that there's a small chance that you may come out of it paralysed,' said the doctor.

Paralysed?

Buggery bollocks!

'Paralysed?' I said.

'Only a small chance,' the doctor replied. 'A very small chance, but a chance.'

Apparently the deep intravenous thing they would have to pierce me with, plus all the chemicals that would be pumped into it, had left some people paralysed.

So that really was that. There was no way on earth I was going to get into a machine a Tourettist and come out of it a paralysed one. No way at all, even if it was for the most laudable and, I'm sure, vital-to-Tourette's-research purposes. Call me selfish, but I'm sorry, I'm just not *that* generous.

CHAPTER 20

SO CLOSE TO SUCCESS

The Prozac kicked in, and I became less anxious about my Touretty tics. There was no radical or marked personality explosion as there had sort of been with the Seroxat, I suppose because there was no more personality in me to burst forth. The Seroxat had helped me over a seemingly impossible hurdle, and helped me to grow into someone who accepted Tourette's as a way of life, someone who no longer fought against it and was able to get on with its normal ups and downs. The Prozac simply helped me regain what had become equilibrium in my busy little world. In other words, I was back again to enjoying a mental dividing line between me and the Tourette's, where we coexisted. It was a situation that I accepted out of necessity. It was the best I could hope for.

The trick of course, since concentration alleviated the tics, was to keep my busy body very busy. I took all the students who came my way, I started teaching piano four days a week in a school with a particularly thriving music department. I did all the examining that was thrown my way, and travelled the length and breadth of the country judging music festivals. I had occasional teaching work at the Royal College, and played concerts whenever and wherever I was asked, just to keep a hand in with my own performance. At home, I practised wildly and socialised almost frantically. It was go, go, go, and I needed it like a drug. In fact, it *was* my drug, the only drug available to me to keep my greedy tics and things at bay.

My tics of course didn't consider my social life to be work, so they sometimes revved up, but I was spending time with one or other of my three closest friends, Alan, Will or Amber, and *they* didn't give two hoots whether I jumped, gyrated, nodded, blinked, blew raspberries or yelped at them. In fact, most people I knew, and still know now, maintain that although they are obviously aware of my Tourettisms on one level, an almost psychological one, they never seem to register or get in between us on a personal level. I suppose people get used to me, and ironically the more I get to know someone, the less on guard I am with my tics. I stifle them less and, in a funny kind of way, feel more at ease. I also learnt to have fun with my tics, bizarre as that may sound. Many a time Alan and I collapsed in hysterics when, halfway through one of our piano duets, I stopped playing completely and went for his nose or ears with all ten fingers. Many a time would Amber's tears of sorrow, during one of her tales of woe, turn into tears of laughter when, midway through one of her most painful confidences, I'd blow a mammoth raspberry.

People in the know also used to make particular sounds, or touch something with all ten fingers, knowing for certain that I'd ape the noise or have to mirror their touch. I'd developed this mimicking thing, you see, and if someone did a certain something, I sometimes had to repeat the action or sound. Apparently this is a common symptom of Tourette's and is called 'echopraxia'. It's also labelled under the echolalia umbrella. My friends had great fun with it.

Will persuaded me to enter an international piano competition. 'You could very well win,' he said. I was dubious about competing at that level. The festivals I judged consisted of people enjoying music-making and performing, and the competitive aspect was there only to add a bit of bite and make the candidates give their best. But international piano competitions, well, I'd heard stories – corruption, sex, bribes, blatant vote-rigging – and I knew that music, or piano playing, can't really be judged on a competitive basis. As I said before, it's not a race, it's subjective. Still, I didn't see the harm in having a go, so I applied. This particular piano competition was in Spain and I quite fancied the idea of playing the piano and getting to eat some authentic tapas and paella. All applicants were screened for their suitability and standard, the competition brochure said, and would be informed by mail whether they had been accepted. It was *so* music profession. So typical. Screenings. Selections. How they screened entrants I really didn't know. They might have hired a private detective to listen to me practising, for all I knew.

So, as well as teaching, examining, adjudicating and giving the odd concert, I now had to prepare the stipulated repertoire for each round of the competition. It was a bit of a bugger really, because there I was practising for the final round of four when, in all probability, I'd be eliminated in the first, as piano competitions are rather like lotteries. But it was good for me, not only for the busyness that I needed to calm me, but also because I'd long forgotten how it felt to be striving, really pushing towards a goal, even a probably unattainable one.

The weeks before the competition flew by and I don't think my Tourette's knew what had hit it, so hard was I working, so happy and busy was I keeping my tics. I would sometimes practise until 2 am and then take the long climb up to the very top of the house and my bed. I'd be up next morning at 6 am and get in a few hours' practice before driving off to teach or examine, or whatever.

Anyway, I ended up in Spain, managed to find a hotel near the competition venue and install myself in a practice room at the music conservatory. However, I was so well prepared that I didn't bother putting in too many hours. All the other competitors were practising away furiously, and when I went to get a coffee and smoke a cigarette, there wasn't a soul in sight, just one massive cacophony of a hundred or so pianos all playing at once. It was rather eerie.

Next day I picked out a number from a hat – the order in which we would play in the competition was determined this way. I was number sixty-five and I chose my piano in the auditorium; there were three available. The auditorium was immense – a red, velvet horseshoe with gold trimming, stalls and three tiers. I tried chatting to some of my fellow competitors but they all seemed so earnest and intense, and they all stuck together in little groups according to their nationalities. There was a gaggle of Japanese girls and a lot of very austere-looking Russians, but I was the only pianist from the

UK, so I stood alone. Forget this, I thought, and decided to take myself off to have some sangria and tortilla in a dusty little taverna. I had to wait two days until it was my turn to play, and during these I must have practised for no more than an hour, as I really didn't want to spend more time than was strictly necessary in the land of the so very serious.

On the day of my first, and probably only, round, I walked onto the platform at exactly 3.17 pm. There was an audience of about two or three hundred. The jury, which consisted of nine eminent musicians, sat in a row alone on the first tier and, as I looked up, I could only make out the tops of their heads. I sat down at the piano and started to play, and, my God, did I play. I even surprised myself. I was so lost in the music that it was almost as though I forgot it was me who was playing it. It was almost like the proverbial out-of-body experience, where you look down and see yourself being you. I played four works in that first round and, for one of a handful of times in my life, I was back to being the lonely little boy miming on his grand piano to records of the great masters, except now it was really me playing. Suddenly I seemed to jump back to reality and realised that I was playing the final notes of my thirty-minute programme. As my hands thundered down to the bottom of the piano I started to wonder if the audience would actually clap for me, and, before my last note had even faded away, my question was answered. Applause rained down on me. I stood to take a bow and there were wolf whistles and yells from the audience, and as I looked up to the jury they were all clapping; one of them even shouted, 'Bravo.' I couldn't believe it. Backstage, people clambered around me, and even other competitors offered their congratulations.

As a result of my performance, I was placed a likely contender for the first prize in the competition, but, as the competition progressed, it became clear that I was not to have such an easy ride after all.

I decided to use some of the time allocated for practice in order to get things tip-top for my forthcoming performances. And I really did practise this time. I went over everything again and again in my most obsessive Touretty, touchy way. There was no room for error, technically or musically. Clarity of mind was what was needed, and was exactly what I had on that first day of practice. But during the night before my second day of practice, I was tormented by nightmares in which I was back at school with everyone laughing at me, spitting at me, teasing and terrifying me. And they weren't just calling me Freaky and Noddy and Blinker, they were yelling about the competition: 'Freaky's going to stop halfway through his performance.' 'Freaky's going to stop.' 'Stop playing, Noddy, stop playing.' I kept waking soaked in sweat, and each time I tried to sleep I'd be woken by the taunting in my head, the same jibes, again and again.

The following day I was a wreck. So much for clarity of mind. I was traumatised. 'It's just pre-competition nerves and pressure,' I kept telling myself. But I didn't believe it. I didn't feel in the least bit nervous or pressured. I wasn't scared of performing, in fact, I was loving it and dying to perform again. So why was I feeling so scared? I dragged myself to practice that day, but never got down to any real work because an old friend popped by to visit. That old friend goes by the name of Touretty and his second name is Nod. My tics, which had been so satisfied, so occupied and contented with all my hard work and performing, decided to send Noddy to pay a visit. And he stayed. I nodded and I nodded and then I nodded more. I was beside myself. I felt that any minute I might nod my neck right out of joint, if such a thing was possible. I sat in my practice room and begged Noddy to go away. To add to it all, I kept remembering my dream, and hostile twisted faces kept shooting into my mind's eye. Then I started ticcing verbally, violently – one a second – and then I started forcing myself to hyperventilate. I knew what was going on. I knew only too well, but why now? Why me? I lay down on the practice room floor and willed myself to calm down, but it's Tourette's we're talking about here, all the willing, all the praying, all the stifling in the world won't make it go away when it really decides to get its teeth into me.

I went to bed that night utterly shattered. The dream came back, but this time it was the jury members who were jeering at me. I kept waking up petrified. I'd never had nightmares like that before. What was happening? Was I losing it completely?

Well, next morning, the morning of my performance, I didn't feel remotely rested, and, as I showered and got dressed, my tics had a field day. They wiped the floor with me. I was to perform at 12 noon for almost an hour, and as I warmed up backstage I started to re-involve myself with my playing again and the tics seemed to subside. But when I got up and went to stand in the wings of the stage, instead of feeling nervous I just stood there nodding and nodding. God only knows what anyone watching me must have thought.

As soon as I walked onto that stage, my tics went scuttling back to wherever it is they live in my brain, and I was fine. I was on. The performance had begun.

I played my heart out. I played for all I was worth and, as before, floated up somewhere and saw and listened to myself as I milked every note from the magnificent instrument. And then it happened. I was no longer somewhere up there, but lucidly in my head, feeling the heat from the lights, feeling my fingers on every single note. I knew what was coming. I felt it rise up, like a warm heat, through my whole body. I felt its gush of unstoppable power hurtling towards my head. I nodded. And then I nodded again. I had *never* nodded or ticced in performance. 'Noooooooooooo,' I screamed silently. My brain kicked in, my musical safety net caught me, and my fingers went onto autopilot and carried on playing all by themselves. *No. Please. Not now.* It was then that everything seemed to speed up in my head. I nodded again and rolled my eyes hard back in their sockets. I remembered my dream and saw those hideous faces. I was nodding and ticcing and blinking and thinking, and then my hands flew up and stayed suspended in mid-air. And I stopped.

There was a gasp from the audience, a murmuring, and I just sat there. A voice from the balcony said, 'Please. Nicholas. Please continue. Please.' But I couldn't. I stood up and walked off, and, by doing so, disqualified myself from the competition. It was over.

There was mayhem backstage. An usher came running up to me and said, 'The chairman of the jury wants you to go back. Go and play. He says it's OK'. I walked past her and pushed my way through a fire exit that led to the street outside. I needed air. I was shaking all over. I started walking, walking anywhere, but voices called to me. I looked back and the sight I saw would have, under normal circumstances, made me guffaw my socks off. There was a train of people moving towards me, competition ushers in red jackets, shuffling Japanese girls, a photographer, some Russians and, to top it all, three jury members. They all stood around me in a circle. 'What happened?' 'Go back.' 'Play.' 'It's OK.' 'Why?' 'Did you forget it?' 'Come on.' 'Go back.' 'Play.' 'Why?' And on and on.

But it was truly over, and I left Spain the following day.

OK, Tourette's. You win. Happy now?

Chapter 21

Burning Bridges

Back in London I found it hard to explain to everyone what had happened to me in Spain. I just told people I'd stopped and that's all there was to it. But *I* knew. I knew why I'd stopped. I hated myself. I despised myself. I hated all that was Touretty me. I hated the doctors who couldn't cure me. I hated and hated and hated.

I withdrew into myself. Despite being on Prozac, which is supposed to be the miracle anti-depressant, I was down. I was negative, angry and devastated. People, my parents, Alan, Amber, Will, kept saying, 'It could have happened to anyone.' But they were wrong. It could *not* have happened to anyone. For most people, most 'anyone's, do not have Tourette's. True, anyone, any pianist can have stage fright, or a memory lapse, or suffer some inexplicable technical failure, but I hadn't. My memory had been fine, my fingers had been in their best form ever and I had not suddenly developed stage fright. 'That's shit,' I wanted to say. 'That's absolute crap. You just don't understand.' But I didn't. They all meant well.

The tics were back with a vengeance and I let them play every dirty little trick in the book on me. 'You can't hurt me anymore,' I told them. 'Do whatever you want, bastards.' I was numb to it all. I didn't give a flying fuck.

Professionally, I worked myself into another frenzy again. It was my escape. I started teaching piano in schools five days a week and giving private lessons at home in the evenings and over weekends.

'He's overtired,' my mother said.

'He's rundown,' my father said.

'You're overdoing it,' my friends said.

But I went on doing it, on and on.

The school year ended and I decided and go to stay with Susanna in Portugal for a month. I needed a break. I desperately needed to escape.

Susanna lives about thirty minutes from Lisbon, in a pretty seaside town called Cascais. It's a lazy place where the sun beats down mercilessly and the sharp sea breeze invigorates the senses. I stayed in Susanna's house without really venturing out for a whole week, sleeping, dozing under an umbrella in her garden and drinking wonderful fruity Portuguese wine by night while chatting to Susanna. She accepted, truly and wholeheartedly accepted, who and what I was years ago. She could tell I was exhausted beyond measure, she knew of my devastating competition performance, although not the details, and she knew I was unhealthily working myself sick. But she never mentioned anything, or pushed me to talk about things. She let me be, and let the conversation go where I wanted it to go. There was no advice and no judgement. Susanna is exceedingly eccentric: she's the mistress of the mixed metaphor and throws these wise and *almost* appropriate sayings into almost every sentence. She is effortlessly sexy, with an earthy appeal that seems to awaken lusty thoughts in men of all ages, and she spends hours pontificating about holistic lifestyles, remedies and energies. An avid fan of Portuguese wines, she likes nothing better than cosily ensconcing herself on a cushion-filled sofa, wine glass near to hand. She's great, and her honest approach to living was exactly what I needed. It was also wonderful for me to spend time with my niece, Sasha, who was a feisty six-year-old with a mean temper, yet a curiously intuitive and sensitive side too.

Since my arrival, Susanna had been telling me that I should drive up to Lisbon and get to know the city. I didn't really know Lisbon too well and was a bit reluctant to drive alone, as Portuguese drivers rate as the second most dangerous in the world – according to one statistic I'd read. As it was, I did brave the roads and drove up to Lisbon several times, although I was scared to death by the other drivers tailing me, usually only centimetres from my rear bumper and racing along at most ungodly speeds. Driving in Portugal was about as close to a near-death experience as I'd ever been. But Lisbon itself was remarkable. It's a dusty city, full of secret passageways, hills and staring old ladies, and I spent many wonderful hours exploring. It was in that city where, for the first time in my life, I fell utterly in love. I met my soulmate. Carlo was a stunningly good-looking, wealthy Italian artist who lived as a recluse in a rambling ex-merchant's palace on the outskirts of Lisbon. We met, on one of his rare outings, at a small party thrown by a Portuguese musician whom I had met years earlier. To say we had so much in common would be a massive understatement;

we gelled on both the physical and emotional level as though we had been designed for each other. Gone were the days of obsessive crushes on totally unsuitable people. Gone were the days of desperately searching for a person who didn't seem to exist. The person did exist. This was the real thing.

So I found love. In fact, *it* seemed to find me. I drove to Lisbon every day then. I felt good inside. I felt warm. I felt at peace. I felt all those wonderfully cheesy clichés about love that wouldn't have turned into such wonderful cheesy clichés had they not all been true. I had found someone who believed that a massive hand had placed us both in the right place, at the right time, for us to be together. I was in love with someone who believed in that age-old dictum of love at first sight. 'Love changes everything,' as the song says. And so it did.

After two weeks, right at the end of my holiday, I was certain of two things. One, that this was not just a holiday romance, and, two, I knew I wanted to move – relocate, pack and up to Lisbon. I knew I would.

Life in London became interminable. I was back to my old work, work, work schedule, yet constantly pining for Carlo. We spoke daily on the phone, but it just wasn't enough. My tics decided to give me a bit of a break and went into a sort of near hibernation, at least while I worked, and they only really popped out to play half-heartedly while I was not working. I went back to Lisbon for weekends, and my love, our love, strengthened as we laughed, loved, listened to music together and explored each other's personalities. For the first time in my life I felt safe enough to let someone close to me, to see me as I really am, to experience that huge and absolutely fundamental part of me that makes me a

Tourettist. And, instead of being rejected as had been my lifelong fear, I was embraced and accepted, loved more even, for being so different.

Back to London – work. Back to Lisbon – love. I was always on the move. Backwards and forwards. Up in the air, then down again. With my lover, then not.

By Christmas I'd given in my notice to the schools where I'd been teaching, I'd cleared my calendar of examining and adjudicating and I'd packed my worldly goods into crates ready for shipping. I was tired of working myself into the ground just to relieve myself of my Tourette's. I was tired of being paid so little for my efforts. I was over it all. I was ready for a change. I needed a new life.

Reading this, it probably looks as though I was committing professional suicide, that I was opting myself out of the music profession, that I was severing my links with the things that many people try so hard to achieve, and that is certainly the view my parents and many other people upheld. 'Jobs like yours don't come easily,' my mother said. 'You're losing all your security,' my father said. 'You'll burn all your bridges,' someone else said.

But that's not how I viewed it at all. I was not blinded by love, or on this occasion madly obsessed. I wasn't *that* naive. I didn't see anything wrong with relocating, or striving for something new. If I'd been deeply satisfied with my career as it was, if I was all set for a glowing future, then I might have been acting stupidly. But there was no prospect of a glittering career, just one that consisted of pretty much the same as I already had, and that was certainly nothing much to write home about. I enjoyed some of it, for sure – the examining, the adjudicating – but spending the rest of my days patiently smiling as under-practised students struggled their way through the most elementary piano pieces, was just not for me. I don't decry the many people who are contented with that, but for me, it would never be enough. I suppose I was basically a frustrated pianist, one whose years and years of dedication to music had left him equipped and experienced enough to play anything or anywhere, but whose sole audience comprised the four deaf walls of his music room. I knew I would never have the performing career of which I had dreamed. I knew I would never be happy until I created a life where my frustration was no longer an issue. So I left. I moved. I started a new life.

The great thing about Portugal was that on my savings, and with help from Carlo, I was able to lead a great life without having to worry about finding work or urgently discovering a niche. Well, for a while.

I lived alone in the centre of the old city, and adapted to not living around other people as though I'd been made for it.

For two years my life was bliss. I wallowed in music, baked in the sun and spent glorious times with my lover. My Tourette's was under control and seemed to appreciate the warmth of the climate. I had feared that the stress of relocating, paired with the shock of suddenly having time on my hands, not being constantly on the go, would trigger one of my bad tic cycles. But it didn't. I still ticced, but my Tourette's seemed happy because I lived alone, somewhere where I was able to give one gala tic variety performance after another, knowing that no one would ever see or hear. I was able to spend hours looking in the mirror, examining every imperfection of my face and body, wondering why I thought, why I was told from inside, that I was so ugly, when I knew that I wasn't at all.

Being in a proper relationship for the first time was something of a learning curve in Touretty terms. Through such close interaction I was learning things about myself, some of which I liked, but many of which I really didn't. I was finding that I was horrendously impatient with Carlo, always thinking I knew the end of sentences, and always bursting for us both to function at my dizzy pace. I saw every argument as a catastrophe, as the beginning of the end and as a seemingly irreparable rift. I obsessed that we were drifting apart when in reality we were doing nothing of the kind. Carlo was learning about Tourette's and about me as a Tourettist, seeing me at my ticcy worst, loving me at my witty best and feeling for me when my barriers fell down and I was overwhelmed with the busy body I have never managed to tame. We also learnt to have fun with my Tourette's, to laugh at situations and events that were blatantly tragic, but which could be diffused by laughter. His demeanour is somehow not that of a typical 'Latino' – not bursting with amiable and immediate warmth – but more one of refinement and control. He always says, that in character, I am the more Latin of the two of us, being more fiery and, at least at face value, more sociable and openly warm. It was a strange balance of personalities that really seemed to work, because underneath our 'external' characteristics, we seemed to fuse into a complete unit, one that discovered peace, security and a comfortable and comforting equilibrium.

We both adored music, live performance and especially opera. But opera performances are not frequent events and, in order to satisfy our craving, we travelled (and still do) to opera houses around the world – Vienna, New York, Berlin, Dresden. Munich, Madrid and London. We stayed in the grandest hotels and ate in the most acclaimed restaurants. We were no sooner back from one trip, than we were getting ready for the next. It was a spoilt and wonderful life, one in the cultural fast lane, and one that we both absolutely relished.

In order to ground myself when not on the go with Carlo, I decided I needed some sort of project in which to immerse myself. I made up my mind to write a book about music with a close Portuguese friend – a new type of guide of a kind that had never been produced before. I spent weeks, months and what spread into years researching and writing, trying to explain classical music in a way that would hopefully turn people on to it, and not away from it. The endless research, combined with collaborating on content with my co-author, provided a goal to work towards and, once again, some professional aspirations.

There were hiccoughs along the way, however. They started after I'd been in Lisbon for two years and began a cycle of mishaps that would result in near tragedy.

CHAPTER 22

DEATH AT THE DOOR

The first hiccough was, of course, Tourette-related. I was heavily obsessing again, thinking violent thoughts and toying with the idea of dangerous behaviour. And then my tics went bananas. It all came on so suddenly. One day I was OK, quite literally ticcing along in my usual merry way, and the next day I was a wreck. Something instinctively told me that the Prozac, which I still took religiously, was doing something to me. What it was doing I didn't know, but my gut told me that it was wrong. That feeling in itself then became an obsession. I rapidly stopped the Prozac and braved horrendous withdrawal symptoms just to get off the damn thing. But I'd been wrong. I didn't rapidly get better. If anything, I got worse. What to do? I tried to find out if there was a doctor in Lisbon, or even in Portugal, who dealt with Tourette's, but no one had heard of it, which seemed strange to me, because I'd seen so many Portuguese people displaying very blatant signs of Tourette's.

So I went back to London to try and see my consultant, or any consultant. But I couldn't get an appointment either through the NHS or privately.

I stayed in London for a whole month trying to get an appointment to see someone who could possibly help me. My parents were at their wits' ends seeing the terrible state I was in and being helpless and unable to alleviate things for me.

As it was, I finally managed to get an appointment at the hospital with a member of the consultant's team. She was a very amiable Yugoslavian lady, and decided that I should try a new type of pill, an anti-depressant called Efexor. She said she had conferred with the main consultant and he too thought it was the best option. I was willing to try anything and happily agreed to give it a go.

I returned to Lisbon and my life. The Efexor calmed me down, and my busy body soon became less busy. I settled back into familiar old patterns, writing, enjoying music, relishing love and gleefully planning trips.

My mother came to stay with me for a few weeks and I enjoyed her eccentricities, her sharp wit and her contagious sense of fun. She was relieved that I seemed so much better with my Tourette's and that I was actually finding my new life rewarding. Just at the end of her stay it was Mother who helped a new hiccough surface. We were lounging on my terrace in the glorious August sun, when I asked her to spray some sun lotion on my back. As she was spraying, she prodded my back, about ten centimetres above my waist-line. 'What's that?' she asked. 'It's weeping.'

Well, I had a feel about and could indeed detect something. I twisted in front of a mirror to get a look and saw a raised sore, or lesion, which was red and seeping clear fluid. Not a spot, I thought. Not a blister. So what is it?

Mother left the next day and I promised I'd see a doctor. Actually I did manage to see one that very day.

'Looks like skin cancer,' he said.

Skin cancer.

I was told that I should have surgery immediately to remove the lesion. Waiting would be dangerous, he said. Thoughts ran through my head: *Private surgery. Private hospital. Big bill. Oh God.*

So I flew back to London and went to see my GP. She peered at my lesion under a magnifying glass and said I must go the emergency lesion clinic. Now. *Oh boy.* The emergency lesion unit receptionist took my doctor's letter, didn't even give it a glance, and said, 'I'll put you on a list. Three to six months.'

Three to six months?

'Is that an emergency appointment?' I asked.

'Yeah,' she said in a bored tone.

'Is this the only emergency lesion clinic I can go to?' I asked.

'Yeah,' was the response again.

'But I might be *dead* in three to six months,' I said.

'Yeah,' she said.

I didn't know what to say, or what to do, and, furthermore, I was fighting a growing urge to spit in the receptionist's left eye. It was so big, like the rest of her, so open and just, well, so *there.*

I grabbed my letter from her fist and said 'Forget it.' And that was the new improved National Health Service? What a joke.

*

That night, as I was trying to get my head around things and wondering what to do, I got a phone call from a friend. It was bad news. My friend Will was dead. There were no details. In fact, no one seemed to know very much at all. Apparently, Will had been on holiday on some Spanish island and had just collapsed, and died a few days later. Even when I managed to speak to his family many weeks later, they still had no clear idea why Will had died. I was devastated. I went and sat in my room and thought about my friend, and tried to make it sink in that he wasn't there any more. I sat and I ticced wildly in fury. Things just weren't fair.

I never did find out why Will died, and I'm still upset that I hadn't been able to go to his funeral in Northern Ireland because I had been dealing my own health problems. I still think about him every day, and regret that I wasn't near him when he faced a journey that I'm certain he wasn't prepared for.

. I had to have private surgery after all. On examination, the lesion had indeed been malignant and, I was told, rather dangerous. There would be no more sunbathing for me ever again.

I returned to Lisbon again, to resume my life. I was responding well on the Efexor, my Touretty tics and state of mind were calm, and I was able to get back to my own little sense of normality. My relationship was still going well and my book about classical music was coming along nicely. Money was running low, though, so I advertised for some private students and managed to get three. Susanna saw a job advertisement in the Portuguese English newspaper. One of the top international schools, located just outside Lisbon, needed a part-time teacher of music. I applied and, although

I was reluctant to start teaching in an institution again, I thought that this one might be rather nice. The school was set in an idyllic location right on the seafront, in a historic building, and I already knew several of its teachers through Susanna. The English community in Portugal all seem to know each other.

The job was offered to me and I started teaching a music class, which was rather fun. It was certainly much more rewarding trying to instil a bit of music into an enthusiastic group, than it was spending half an hour with an under-practised brat. I had been a little concerned that I might give myself away as a Tourettist. Having experienced first-hand that cruel streak that children have, I was dead scared that I might tic in class and lay myself open to potential ridicule and open up old wounds. But that didn't happen. I may well have been unable to stifle the odd tic in my classroom, but I don't think the kids ever caught on.

I got on famously with the majority of staff at the school, but a small few kept well clear of me for some reason, and I wondered if being in an institutional setting again somehow made me give off those 'arrogant' or 'pushy' vibes that had so obviously marred my Royal College days. By and large things went very smoothly, though. I managed to disguise my Tourettisms and I enjoyed the colourful interaction of working in an international school. Apart from the occasional run-in with administration and those in authority, which I put entirely down to the directness of my Tourette's and not to bad intention, the experience was a very agreeable one.

By contrast, I was starting to develop this overreaction thing in my relationship. It began to provoke hideous rifts, and not only a lot of confusion, but also a great deal of resentment on both sides. I would take offence at the smallest and often most insignificant things and blow them completely out of proportion. I'd quite literally erupt, and scream, kick and shout. I was having tantrums. When my short-lived fury subsided and when I couldn't see what all the fuss had been about, that was the point when Carlo tended to launch into me for my previous overreaction. It was stalemate time and time again.

Ever since my relocation to Portugal, I had been getting closer to Susanna. I had taken to spending the weekends with her and her small family. Sasha, my niece, was still at that wonderful age when everything is so fascinating, and I loved chatting with her, having to leave the baggage of my own life behind, as I met her on that wonderfully naive and magical emotional plane where everything, in her view, was so possible. I also explained to her what Tourette's is, how it affected me and why it made me do funny things. I remember her listening intently, as she did her best to meet me on my rather more serious plane. She studied me thoughtfully for a moment, and my eyes filled with tears as she said, 'I know you're not like everyone else. It makes me love you even more.'

All hell broke loose when my parents decided to sell their London house and move to Portugal for a trial period. They were both retired now and wanted to be near me and Susanna. There were big plans to embrace a new way of life, enjoy some outdoor living and a more clement climate. But while they were going through the upheavals of packing and waving their goodbyes to London, my life fell apart.

I had developed a nagging pain, an ache, deep in my abdomen, and I was worrying, speculating furiously and obsessing over what it might be.

I was still working hard and trying to keep my busy body occupied. But the pain didn't go away, it continued to nag. I tried to work out if my tic – the one where I pull my stomach in as tightly as possible, hold, and then push it out with a painful straining – was making me ache. Was I doing myself some sort of damage, or was the tic actually damaging me?

Susanna had become my closest confidante and I told her my health worries. I speculated like crazy – is it the stomach tic that's doing it? Could it be HIV or AIDS, although that would be incredibly unlikely? Was it a tapeworm literally eating me from the inside out? I was starting to lose weight. *What if . . . could it be . . . maybe . . . is it?* And on and on.

I secretly took a day off school and went to see a doctor. He wasn't particularly impressed by my symptoms, but nonetheless ordered a CAT scan and a comprehensive series of blood tests, which I suffered reluctantly because I was so syringe phobic, something that probably stemmed from a little discovery I'd made when I was a child, when I'd been rummaging through Jeremy's room, and found two syringes streaked inside with blood that he'd obviously used to inject heroin.

In the week when I had to wait for a phone call from the doctor with the test results, my Tourette's went crazy again. It must have been the stress and worry, and it was certainly the obsessing, that did it. My mind kept going over things and possibilities again and again, and I somehow started to rehash old tics that I thought had left my Touretty memory long ago. It was yet another example of the selfishness of the syndrome and the way it attacks me more furiously when I'm trying to focus on something else.

I got a call from the doctor the following week and he told me I'd better make an appointment immediately, and, with mental alarm bells deafening me, I dashed off to see him.

With a look of dread on his face, he sat behind his desk and delivered the news.

'It's cancer,' he said. 'Lymphoma.'

I couldn't speak.

'It's aggressive,' he continued. 'You need to start treatment immediately and I'll arrange everything for you.'

Cancer? Treatment? Aggressive?

No, that's not possible. It's just not possible.

I didn't know what to say. My mind was a jumble. I suppose I should have asked for medical specifics, or a second opinion, or what sort of treatment he meant, but I couldn't.

'Will I die?' I finally managed to ask.

'Maybe,' he said.

CHAPTER 23

RADIOACTIVE TOURETTE'S

My head was spinning. It was strange, because in between having been told that I had lymphoma and actually starting treatment, I seemed to feel more unwell by the day. I'm not sure if it was because of real symptoms, or whether I, my body, had reacted to the news and psychosomatically decided to make itself ill. Nonetheless ill is what I was. Ill and terrified. I didn't tell anyone except Susanna, and I swore her to secrecy. In any case, I didn't know how to go about telling people – my family, friends and Carlo. I didn't want everyone to suddenly bustle around me, even if the bustling would be from good intentions. I didn't want people to start mourning me before I'd even died or at least had the chance to put up a bloody good fight. I knew that death was a possibility, where, when or how I didn't know exactly, but somehow I felt it lurking in my shadow.

My parents had just moved to Portugal, and were living near Susanna in Cascais. Their move from London, after a whole life there, had been particularly traumatic, and, now that the move was over and they were settling in to their new life, they decided that they didn't want to be there after all. They were miserable in Portugal and frantic with worry that they had made a huge and irreversible mistake. Susanna tried to help them as much as she could, and, in normal circumstances, I too would have been around to lend a hand or an ear. But I was conspicuously absent and my parents started getting miffed. They'd moved to Portugal to be near their children and I was nowhere to be found. You see, I just couldn't visit them. I couldn't face them. I was constantly making excuses that I hoped seemed valid to them. I gave up my teaching job immediately; I couldn't even work through a notice period. The doctor hadn't been joking when he told me to be prepared for a long and consuming fight, so I cleared my life of any obligations and prepared for whatever it was that life had decided to throw at me now.

It all seemed so futile. Battling my way through school, fighting my tics, trying to overcome my obsessions and compulsions, conquering my low self-esteem, slogging away at the piano, battling against the desire to spit in people's eyes, trying not to touch every greasy nose that whetted my touching appetite, dealing with malignant skin cancer and now having to put my shields up, muster all the strength I had to wage war on lymphoma; cancer with great, big, fat C. I wondered what the hell it was all about. Did I live just to fight? I didn't want to fight any more. I felt like crawling under my duvet and going into denial about the whole bloody thing, my whole miserable 'fight, fight, fight and then fight again' life.

And that's exactly what I did. I turned my phone off, closed all the shutters, told everyone I had flu, lay in darkness, curled up in my bed and stayed there for two whole days, only surfacing to go to the bathroom or sip some water. I slept and I thought. I replayed my life over and over again. I put every possible ending to every single scenario, and imagined how things might have been had I chosen different paths. I wondered if in the end all routes would lead me to exactly the same place. I lay there and imagined what death would be like, whether it would be just a black nothingness, or whether I'd have to endure more obstacles on the other side and fight again. I wondered if anyone would really care, if anyone would remember me, or if I'd just fade into the past and become a distant memory of a guy who spent his whole life fighting Tourette's, building a life and then having it destroyed by cancer. I realised that I was nothing. All my dreams of being a world-acclaimed pianist, all those dreams of making a mark, of doing something that really mattered, all those dreams that had never been realised, would die with me and no one would ever know that I had even had them, or that I'd once strived for someone to hear my little message. I cried and I laughed. I relived moments when I had made a difference, when people had been touched by my performance, and I felt their applause, I heard it and I knew that I would never hear it again. I gave up.

And then a peculiar thing happened. I had been asleep for about fifteen hours, woke with a start, jumped out of bed and said, 'Fuck this for a game of soldiers, I'm NOT giving up.' As I showered, dressed and ate, I kept saying over and over again, 'Come on, pull yourself together, go and show them what you're made of.' I felt rejuvenated. I was ready. I could endure.

I started radiotherapy, and no sooner had it begun than I was back to feeling beaten again emotionally. So much for my endurance. It was a mind-destroying routine. Wake up, go to the hospital, get zapped, go home, feel like shit, go to bed and then do it all the next day, again and again, on and on. I had the weekends off and lay around like a cabbage, unable to brave seeing anyone, and too weak to even try.

I managed to pull myself together enough to see Carlo for dinner a couple of times a week, but, since my heart wasn't in it, I suppose I started to give out strange vibes. I was tense and more easily upset than usual. We bickered and fought. I started losing my temper and began my old overreacting-at-the-slightest-thing routine. Carlo still had no idea what I was going through, what I was dealing with, as I had still not let the cat out of the bag. But with every day that passed, I knew that I was going to eventually have to tell someone other than Susanna. I knew I'd have to tell everyone. It was too much for me to bear alone anymore. I couldn't keep the act up for much longer as I was looking more drawn by the day, had great big purple welts under my eyes and was losing weight by the kilo. Everyone expected me to be my normal self, and I just couldn't act my part.

My Tourette's, inconsiderate as it is, didn't decide to help me out a bit by easing off even slightly. Actually, I think all the radiation it was getting went to its (my) head. I went through practically my whole Touretty repertoire, the one that had begun when I was seven and developed and mutated over the years, over and over again. As if I wasn't exhausted enough already, I had to jump in the air, punch my tender stomach, jerk my neck, nod, roll my eyes, yelp, hoot and all the rest, all of the other spiteful and exhausting things that made me the Tourettist I was. But now the tics somehow felt different. That welling up of energy, the absolute order to tic or do whatever Touretty thing I had to do, seemed more focused, even more direct than usual, maybe even almost more identifiable. Instead of just being aware of the whoosh of energy surging through my body prior to a tic, it now felt as though it was part of the tics and not just a prelude. I felt that energy welling up and releasing itself as though it was boiling hot water shooting out from somewhere around the region of the mythical solar plexus and moving up towards my brain where it would then make me tic. It was unequivocally spectacular, tumultuously energising and almost enough to make me reel, as though some wonderful recreational drug had just been injected into a main artery.

This went on for days on end, and then it would cease and the welling-up thing would go back to normal. I can only assume that it was because of the radiation, because of the drugs. The doctors had said that I would have side effects, so I suppose my old enemy from within was doing just that and reacting. I had hoped that the Tourette's and the cancer might somehow have cancelled each other out – each inadequacy attracting the other, thus merging into an unidentifiable something that gave me some relief. Naively, I thought that the two 'deficiencies' might find their own symmetry and get along nicely and, hopefully, without me. But they never did. Tourette's and cancer somehow became enemies within me, and I was the battleground on which each launched their most destructive weapons.

Eventually, I had to tell my parents. I couldn't hold it back from them any longer. My mother went into shock and, for the first time in my life, I thought that she was about to throw in her towel. But then she revved all her engines, and fought and battled with me. She was positive and did all she could to make my life stress-free. She had lost one son, she said, and she had no intention of losing another. She willed me to fight, to live, and her strength often tided me through great long periods when I thought that I had none of my own left. My father, who is deaf and constantly dealing with his own inner battles, took a slightly more negative view initially. He kept saying, 'I'm losing another son,' which didn't really help me much since I thought there was probably a good chance that he might actually be right. Having said that, I had to appreciate that his life had been torn apart. He was clinically depressed, and I think suffered some sort of nervous breakdown through the move from London not living up to his expectations.

So my father was depressed, my mother was dealing with my father and simultaneously trying to find a new house in London for them to buy in order to move back, Susanna was trying to balance concern for my parents against the running of her own family with its own ups and downs, and they were all devastated, yet willing me on in my own battle. It was all a complete mess.

And then I told Carlo. I had support and love there and I knew it. I wasn't abandoned because I was sick, or avoided because death was knocking at my door, I was just loved, and love is exactly the thing that I needed most. Love was what would get me through. Love would cure me, or so I hoped. Love from my family, from Carlo and from my close friends. I was losing everything, in fact I felt as though I had lost everything, but I never lost love.

I still lived alone; my family said that I should move in with them so they could be there for me, but I didn't want to. It was enough for me to know that people were there for me, but I needed my space. I needed privacy. I needed to just be. The fight was mine, and, with the best will in the world, no one else could help me, or join me on my bumpy ride. I was just so lucky to have so much support, both emotional and financial. Despite the severity of my illness, I was for a very long time in the privileged position of not having to worry about matters financial, which was a huge burden lifted from me. My parents and Carlo made sure that bills were paid on time, that I had money for whatever was needed and that I wanted for nothing.

I decided to order a new piano in the hope that the excitement and joy it would give would help to ease my burden. I had visions of turning to music as my saviour as I always had in the past, of playing my way through my misery. But when the piano arrived I had no strength to play it. I sat and looked at it, sometimes for hours. In my head I heard the music it should have been playing. I longed to hear it, but I couldn't go near it. It just sat there day after day as a constant reminder of what should have been, and I started to resent it as its casework gleamed invitingly with reflections of light. In the end, I threw a large blanket over it so I wouldn't have to see it staring back at me all day long, unused, unplayed and silent.

I couldn't even listen to music anymore, either. The sounds seemed to hurt my ears and vibrate painfully through a body that was at war with itself. The music that had always been present in my head stopped, and it felt like a massive pause button somewhere in my brain had been depressed. I was suddenly a musical wilderness. I was utterly empty.

Because I wasn't able to eat, my body mass continued to waste away. I had no appetite and felt so wretched from the radiotherapy, and latterly chemotherapy, that I had no desire to eat anything. A friend suggested baby food in the hope that if I managed even a few small pots of it a day I'd at least be getting some nutrients. So I explored all the wonderfully mushy combinations of lamb and peas, chicken and carrots, beef and parsnips, and sat like a great baby playing with the runny combinations, occasionally popping a spoonful in my mouth, but more often than not just staring at tiny pots of food that, despite their jazzy names, tasted like unflavoured mush.

I was on a downer all right. I didn't feel that my treatment was going well, in fact, I knew that it wasn't. The doctors told me that instead of losing its hold on me, the level of lymphoma seemed to be increasing. I had to have some lymph nodes removed from under my arm and I was fast becoming devastated. My doctor told me to double my daily dose of Efexor – the anti-depressant that had been pre-scribed for my Tourette's, but which was now fittingly coming to the rescue for the thing it had actually been produced for. Not that I have ever been a clinically depressed person. Whatever life throws at me, however demoralised I am, I never sink into the absolute abyss of darkness that quite lit-erally seems to permeate and ooze from every cell of a true depressive person.

Taking double didn't really seem to do much for me in any way. It didn't reduce the feeling that I was carrying a heavy burden, because I really was carrying one, and no amount of pills in the world could take away that reality. Nor did the doubling of the Efexor help my Tourette's. My obsessions remained as potent as ever and my tics, if anything, worsened. I was quite literally under attack. A dull, un-locatable and silent attack from lymphoma that I imagined was eating away at me, and a much more flamboyant and verbose one from an attacker called Tourette's. All I wanted to do was rest, but my brain knew better, and I cursed it as it made me go through my paces as a now radioactive Tourettist. Some days I didn't think I could go on anymore, and wondered if I shouldn't just lie down on my bed and say, 'Take me. Go on, you bastards, just do it,' to everything that was eating away at me, chewing painfully at every muscle and every little nerve, making me do things I didn't want to do, demanding more from me, and craving my attention every second, never once having the decency to just let me rest. I hated my Tourette's, loathed myself for having it and despised and resented every little thing it made, forced, ordered me to do.

Now, before I precipitate a mass grabbing for the box of tissues so you can shed a tear for my sorrows, I'm going to close the door on the cancer episode entirely – well, hopefully.

I got through it. It *was* touch-and-go for a while and I had to have lumps and things removed, undergo chemotherapy, lose my hair, whittle my body down to skeletal proportions and all the rest, all for nearly two years. But I made it. The cancer left me.

The Tourette's, of course, didn't.

CHAPTER 24

DRILL SERGEANT

I'd long come to the view that whatever happened, whatever I went through, whichever pills I took, Tourette's would be there. In fact, it has been the only constant in my life, and though there were times when I'd view it as a menace, there were other times when it seemed to stand as the only reminder to me that I was still functioning, that I was alive. It had often been the only tenuous tie left to a life I'd almost given up on.

Despite my natural jubilation on being told that I was in the clear from the cancer, I still found myself on edge. I was continuing to get in a state and overreact generally to the smallest things. OK, I had no job, my money had all but disappeared entirely, I had no real prospects save a few rather hazy ideas or plans, but I felt as though I was carrying the world's problems on my shoulders. I started obsessing over the most ridiculous and irrelevant things, really making a meal out of them. Like going crazy if I had to queue too long in a shop, or losing my temper completely with myself if I had a knot in my shoelaces, or feeling it was the end of the world because I had a great big zit on my forehead. Stupid, really minor things were becoming a big issue for me.

I also began to become somehow more regimented with my tics. If I shook my head it had to be three times, and followed immediately with a hard nod, which then had to be complemented by a hard punch to my stomach, with a mother of a raspberry to round things off. That sort of thing, and countless other variations. My Tourette's had always demanded strange things and I'd often had to comply to a degree of ritualistic behaviour with my tics. But this new, almost military precision, with which I had to execute certain movements and make various sounds, was new simply because it was so dictatorial.

It was like my Tourette's had somehow evolved from being the haphazard, selfish and needy thing that it always was, into a great, burly sergeant major, who was screaming out orders to a drill squad. It wasn't that I was doing a Joan of Arc impersonation and really losing it and hearing orders in my head from an imaginary being, it was more like *I* was the one both giving the orders and obeying them. Where did the line of command stop? Who was calling the shots here? If I was ordering myself to do a certain routine of Tourettisms, then what was ordering me to give myself that order? I had no answers to my own questions, and wondered if I was now dealing with something a lot more serious than just plain old Tourette's. Had I developed some kind of real madness? Was Tourette's just a crazy-paved path that led to lunacy? I was desperately confused and couldn't talk to anyone about it, because I feared they would think me utterly insane. There was no way I was going to see a Portuguese doctor about Tourette's.

I remembered my enquiries before in trying to find someone who could deal with it, when no doctor had ever even heard of TS. I had visions of being locked away in a padded room in a straight-jacket if I saw a Portuguese doctor.

I decided that I'd try quitting the Efexor, after all, I had only doubled the dose because of a depression that had now sort of lifted. Maybe it was overstimulating me. Maybe it was doing more harm than good. Whatever the case, it was clearly not helping anymore. I cut it down by half and nothing happened. I gave it a few weeks, and my tics and the orders to tic, and my Touretty needs and compulsions, stayed pretty much the same. So I decided to come off the Efexor completely, assuming that I could try taking my pill a little later than usual, spreading out the time between doses, and eventually reducing to nothing. That didn't work. Almost to the hour, at the time when my Efexor was due, my body started playing up; I knew it was screaming for the Efexor. It was awful. I'd start to shake, my vision would blur, I'd be lathered in sweat and feel about as nauseous as I'd ever felt before. Shit.

I then became obsessed with getting off the Efexor. I began to feel as though it was smothering me, I felt like a claustrophobic tied up in a ropes and unable to move. It was terrifying. So I started taking a small grain out of each capsule that I took, in the hope that I'd not only be able to wean myself off, but also succeed in fooling my brain into thinking that, since it was still getting a nice little capsule, it was still getting the right dose. Well, that sort of worked. Almost. After about three weeks I was barely taking any Efexor at all, and decided it was time to stop taking it completely. I went to bed, drifted off to sleep and all hell broke loose.

First I started hearing voices, loud voices, shouting at me, over and over again. I'd wake up with a start, tell myself everything was fine and then try to sleep again. And then the dreams started. I was plagued by the most hideous nightmares imaginable, one after another. I'd wake up and feel the relief of being safe, and then realise that I wasn't awake at all – the thing that was out to get me in the previous dream was there waiting for me. I hadn't woken at all, you see. I'd just dreamt that I'd woken. These dreams, these two-layered double dreams, went on all night long, and by the morning I was in a state of near devastation. But I didn't want to take Efexor. I knew that I'd end up weaning myself back onto them if I did that. The day turned out to be almost as bad as the night. No daydreams, but more sweats, more nausea, more blurred vision and then strange visions when, if I turned my head in a natural movement, it seemed as if the things I was seeing in the room were not moving at the same rate as my eyes, but slower, only to 'thud' and lock into correct position when my head, or I, stopped moving.

Then the worst of all, I started having what I latterly found out were called 'brain shocks', or 'brain shivers'. I can't tell you how awful these are. About three times a minute it felt as though an electric current was being passed through my brain, during which time, it seemed to wobble or shiver. I was clucking away like a drug addict desperate to get the next fix.

Meanwhile, my tics and obsessions and orders still kept on coming at me; there was no let-up from anything. Whereas before I'd found peace by sleeping, I was now too scared of potential nightmares to do even that. I used to lie on my sofa and beg, literally plead with the brain shocks and dizziness to stop, pray for my tics to calm down just for a few moments, to give me a break, to just show a bit of mercy on a poor guy who was only trying to get off a pill and go back to a normal, if Touretty, life. 'Please just go away. Please. Please.' But nothing stopped. Not even for a second.

I lasted three days and nights like that and I ended up feeling more shattered from that lack of Efexor than I had ever felt when I was fighting cancer. I went online and browsed the Web, looking for anything that would help me, some advice on getting off Efexor. I was shocked by what I discovered: hundreds and hundreds of posts on forums, with people pleading and imploring for advice on how to get off Efexor. You see, it may be a wonder drug when you are on it, but getting off it was, according to many threads I read in the forums, the hardest thing some people had ever had to do in their lives. I must have sat for five hours reading account after account of dreams, brain wobbles, nausea, panics, sweats, all side effects from withdrawing from Efexor. So what did I do? I literally ran and got my box of Efexor, and I popped two in my mouth. Hey presto, I felt right as rain within fifteen minutes. I felt great, still ticcing away furiously, still jerking away with military precision, still ordering myself to do things, but absolutely A1 fabulous about it.

You might wonder, if I was kind of OK on the Efexor, then why I wanted to go through the hell of trying to get off it. Or, what a futile exercise it was if I only ended up back on it again. But it wasn't a futile experiment for me. I needed to know if the Efexor had been contributing to my latest Touretty developments. Even though I knew that when I had been off it for just a few days my Tourettisms didn't let up, I really don't know if they stayed the same, or how severe they were on my 'normal' scale, because I was trying to deal with the brain shocks and all the things that went with the withdrawal symptoms. I'd been in no position to judge it objectively.

So I remained on the Efexor, feeling almost guilty that I hadn't had the strength to expel it from my life, but also angry that I was on something that now seemed to control me. I was an addict.

I now faced an even larger conundrum. I didn't know what I wanted to do with my life, where I wanted to be or what kind of future I wanted. I found myself staring back at everything that had passed, yet unable to look forward, unable to see myself in the future. I had a loving family, an adoring partner and loyal friends, but as far as I could see, very little else. I suppose somewhere along the way I'd decided that I wanted to do something big, to make people notice me, to make an impact and make a difference. Whether this stemmed from Touretty obsession, a reaction to having been a nobody at school or from sheer vanity, I really didn't know. I hadn't been equipped enough to plough ahead in the world and seek fame and fortune so far, because it seemed I had nothing much to offer anyone. I'd given the piano thing my best shot, given it my life, in fact, but, through no fault of my own, it just hadn't been meant to work out. I supposed that I'd failed. That was the bottom line. I was a great big failure. Everyone kept saying, 'Hold on to your dreams, don't let them go,' or 'You've just spent years fighting cancer, what do you expect,' or 'Go and fight, build a new life.' But in all honesty what could I do? Teach? Go back to the old life I'd once had? Rebuild it all again from nothing? Fight all over again, for so very little? I knew what I didn't want, I really did. But I didn't have a clue what I did want.

As my Tourette's got worse by the day, there was more and more tension in my relationship with Carlo. Hideous grievances began to surface that questioned the whole foundation of everything we'd built up. Massive fights and tension ensued. Somehow it was all slipping away and out of my grasp, rolling down a road that could only lead to separation, and I felt powerless to stop it. One final incident broke the strongest link of our invisible chain of love and sent us both reeling away from each other. I had no way to explain to Carlo that what had happened had, on my part, derived from a self-destructive Touretty obsession that, in itself, stemmed from a compulsion to play with things dangerous to myself. It all started with the familiar old surge of feeling ugly within. I obsessed over ways to convince myself that, one way or another, I was still attractive to others. So I decided to play around on the internet in chat rooms, selling myself to prospective partners as what I knew they wanted me to be. I know many people now use the internet for a quick fix of sexual gratification, whether through a dirty chat or a naughty exchange on webcam, but for me, there was nothing sexually satisfying about my chat room activity. I was in it for the emotional kick, nothing more. It was power play. I even went so far as to meet some of the people with whom I'd chatted, never with the ultimate (and, on their part, expected) aim of actually having physical contact with them, but simply so I could reject them, and, by doing so, feel better about myself. In order to feel I was in control of myself I needed to exert it over others by disappointing them in something I knew they wanted, something I could have given but didn't. It was a dangerous and undeniably stupid game, but one over which I obsessed, and one that became crucial for me. I needed to prove to myself that I was still a desired commodity, not to Carlo, but en masse. It felt good. I felt powerful. This new personal need to justify myself became like a drug and I made 'dates', in the full knowledge that I would get that fabulous feel-good factor from my exploits.

But Lisbon is a small city and one of the most irritating characteristics of the Portuguese seems to be their need for gossip. Word got around. Unbeknown to me, Carlo got to hear of my activities. He heard about my arranged 'dates' and caught me in the act of actually meeting someone. Of course he had no idea that I was not being physically or even emotionally unfaithful. How could he have guessed? He viewed the situation at face value and, to his mind, saw me as being adulterous, which I was certainly not. Anger and hurt overflowed from him like a burst and demented fountain and I had no way of explaining the twisted logic behind my actions, my almost sickening motives, my unnatural desire to paint myself as a normal and attractive product to the world at large. I could find no way to justify my deeds. Words were not enough to describe my inner turmoil, my fight with compulsions and Touretty desires, which creep up on me and end up consuming me. My enemy, the Tourette's, had succeeded in destroying a love that I believed was unbreakable, and I loathed myself all the more.

So I packed my things. My life fitted easily into cardboard packing crates. My piano was sent back to London to my parents' new home. I would bloody well go back, and if anyone wanted to laugh and tell me that I was stupid to have burnt my bridges in the first place, then I would endure their laughter. Somehow I would start over again.

With my life safely boxed, I decided to go and stay with Susanna for a while to see if I could get my head in some sort of working order. It was so what I needed, to be around a family, a really cool family, with no pressure, no expectations and no hard-lined advice. I felt myself healing. My body got stronger, and my mind started to feel more serene. Instead of frantically worrying about the future, and desperately trying to figure out what I'd have to end up doing, I just said to myself, 'I'll find something. Don't force things. The right way will become clear. You'll get through.' Some of my old strength was returning, and even though most it was still being consumed by the never-ending appetite of my tics and other Tourettisms, I was getting my own energy back, the energy that had always managed to get me through whatever was thrown at me.

Chapter 25

Full Circle

I wrenched myself away from the sanctuary of Susanna's home in Portugal and arrived back in London at my parent's place. There were no heralding fanfares for my arrival, no celebratory homecoming parties, just a, 'Well, I'm back,' from me and that was that.

I took a few days to get my bearings again. I caught up with old friends, had long coffee and gossip sessions with Alan and walked familiar streets all over again. It was all rather nice actually.

I still didn't know exactly what it was that I wanted to do with my life, but not knowing felt kind of right. It was almost an exciting feeling, not quite knowing where it was that life was going to take me next and, when it did, if it would be somewhere worth visiting. I suppose that I should have been in a massive panic, a kind of 'What the hell am I going to do?' But I wasn't. If nothing else, life had thus far taught me that planning ahead and relying on things was futile, because all those plans could easily be knocked on the head in a flash. That's not to say I felt bitter or hard done by. Far from it. I just didn't see the point in planning too much.

What was nice was that no one put any pressure on me. I was given a wide berth because I was still, despite feeling OK, recovering from a long fight with lymphoma. People didn't tread ever so gently around me – I would have hated that – but they simply didn't ask too many questions. The last thing I wanted was to be constantly explaining myself to people, justifying why my life in Portugal went so off the rails, how I had lost everything I had worked for and how I felt that I didn't really have much of a future.

In my head, of course – in the few moments of the day when I could actually focus on me without having to focus on what I was being forced to do thanks to Tourette's – I knew that I'd better start trying to get things in order. But doing what? I had no idea. 'Try and get a nice little practice of private students,' my father would say. *Great.* 'Get in touch with old contacts and see if you can get a teaching job,' my mother would say. *Please.* 'How about trying to get some concerts?' a friend would suggest. *As if.* 'Ships again?' *No.* 'A change of career entirely?' *What career?* And on and on.

I knew that people were only trying to be helpful when they made their suggestions, and I made modest noises of appreciation, noises that at least led them to believe I was considering their advice, but I had no intention of actually acting on any of it. Being ill and fighting for survival had led me to wonder what it was all supposed to be about. Life, I mean. I'm just trying to say that having been through what I had, I wasn't going to set off down Compromise Avenue again. Why fight so hard for life if you only end up doing what you never wanted to end up doing in the first place?

It was a little harrowing at first, suddenly being in a place so full of people as London always is. In Portugal, the streets simply do not teem with people day and night as they do here, and I suddenly found myself assaulted again (and again) with so much Touretty temptation. A greasy nose here, an elbow there, a bony knee somewhere, and more things to count, more eyes to (desire to) spit in than I'd seen in a long time. London is temptation city for a professional Tourettist like me and I really had to hold myself back sometimes, as my Touretty mind found itself rejoicing in all the activity and movement.

As a means of escaping, maybe even denying decisions that I knew I'd have sooner or later have to confront, I turned to my oldest friend for company and started playing the piano again. I hadn't touched it for years, because during my cancer I hadn't even had enough energy to lift a finger. When I first sat down to play I must confess that, far from being the nimble-fingered whiz-kid I'd once been, I had about as much digital facility as a baboon with club fists. It was almost heartbreaking, and would have been had I not burst out laughing at my own pitiable efforts and utter incompetence. If I tried to make my fingers move remotely fast they just seemed to sit and stare back at me defiantly, like plump Cumberland sausages on a platter. If I tried to play something smoothly it came out like a lumpy dirge, and when I tried to put my back in to it, put a bit of weight behind my arms to play loudly, then it sounded as though I'd just thrown a leg of lamb at the keyboard. It was unpromising. But, after a few days of serious practise, I did manage to get some of my old dexterity back, which was heartening. But, then again, it was a bit sad that my musical standards had dropped so low.

After I'd been back in the UK for a few weeks, my Tourette's flared up like never before. I suppose it was inevitable, seeing as my repertoire of Touretty things had almost taken a back-seat role since my return to London, what with my having to acclimatise myself all over again. It was shocking at first, then demoralising. All the Touretty things that I did seemed to magnify not only in severity, but also in my perception of them. The old feeling of desperation started to nag at me and I braced myself for another Touretty long haul.

But then something unexpected happened. I was walking along the road, ticcing away as I do, and suddenly one word seemed to hurl itself at me. This word, and everything that goes with it, felt as though it was embedding itself deep into my being and penetrating every aspect of my psyche. Although the word was coming from within, I felt as though I was hearing it, or understanding it even, for the very first time.

Acceptance.

It wasn't like one of those spiritual wake-up calls that we are always hearing about, the sorts of things that supposedly happen in an instant and change people's lives forever. I'm afraid I didn't see a vision, hear a voice, or experience some form of transcendental levitation. Nothing of the kind. What did happen, though, was no less meaningful; I decided it was time to wholeheartedly accept myself and, in doing so, embrace myself as a Tourettist in every sense. It was a moment of unexpected clarity and, perhaps, something that had been floating around in my subconscious for years, trying to reach the surface. Despite my years of fighting the syndrome, trying to 'domesticate' my own body, shut myself up, disguise who and what I really am, I knew, useful and necessary as it had all been, that I had never truly *accepted* it. I'd tried, I'd thought I was accepting, I'd even told myself I was, but the whole concept had never sat comfortably within me.

There is no cure for my syndrome, I do occasionally feel as though I'm existing in a nightmare and I hate having to tic and gyrate like I'm giving some colourful rendition of a tarantella, but, and this is a huge but, it is who I am. It is *what* I am. It was all so simple really, and I wondered why I'd had to endure such a long and agonising journey to get to this point. The unforeseen and entirely new concept of real acceptance came as such a shock to me that I was drained for days, but not unpleasantly so. I felt as though I was being wrapped in soft and comforting velvet, it was like the feeling of peace and tranquillity you get when lying on a deserted beach as the sun goes down. It was like shedding a hair shirt and replacing it with the finest cashmere.

As the days went on, so did this unusual new feeling of composure. Yes, my body still moved to its own beat, I still ticced and blew mega raspberries, I yelped and grimaced, but, instead of stifling it all, I just let it happen. I simply *stopped* stifling. I stopped seeing myself as a sub-person with deficiencies of vast proportions. I stopped hating myself when I caught someone eyeing me suspiciously because of some or other Touretty thing I did, and I found myself eyeing them back with a shrug or a smile. And the great thing about it all was that I didn't have to go through any teething period of finally finding my way in the big world, one small step at a time, because I did the acceptance thing in one huge leap. And there was nothing particularly brave about it either, for I was just being myself.

This new-found glee with myself rapidly led me to approach many things very differently. Most importantly, I started seeing myself once again as someone with something to offer and not just another poor soul written off on life's scrap heap. I even went to the piano and played some of my old party pieces, things I was always able to throw off at the drop of a hat, and I actually enjoyed playing them all again, surprising myself with how good they were after so long. Then, I thought long and hard about my Tourette's treatment options – drug regimens and my dealings with a medical profession that had, for so many years, been a big concern to me. I've tried medicines and approaches galore, desperately wanting them to work. I've fought against nonchalance and indifference from medical specialists who I have all but begged to help me. I've coped with one disappointment after another as things didn't work out. But no more. Never again. No more desperation. New measures were called for.

Out of curiosity of what would happen if I went totally drug free for a while, I decided to find a way of getting off the Efexor without suffering again. The problem was my fear of the withdrawal symptoms – brain wobbles and near emotional collapse – and I was petrified of going through that 'cold turkey' process again. I went to the trusty internet to see if someone, somewhere, had discovered a solution to the Efexor enigma. But no one had. There was only one solution; I would have to seek professional help. I decided to see my family doctor about the conundrum.

I'd been registered at the same surgery since I was a baby and the head of the practice, an astute and kindly doctor of the 'old school', whom I'd first seen about my tics when seven years old, had long retired. His successor – a glamorous and powerfully reassuring lady – brought a positive and upbeat energy to the surgery. She has, over the years, tried so hard to find a way of making life more bearable for me because of my Tourette's and has been consistently supportive. Although she isn't a neurologist, I actually have more faith in her simply because she is so nice about it all. There are no judgements from her, no hard sell of horrid and dangerous anti-psychotic medicines, just a level-headed and decisive approach to doing anything to make me more comfortable. She dealt with my fears with a quick stroke of her pen on a prescription pad, putting me on Prozac to break my Efexor addiction.

I managed an amicable divorce from Efexor and then Prozac, and was finally free of drugs. It didn't feel all that bad, and, other than feeling a bit 'lost', I did pretty well, for a while. The most important thing for me was a feeling of achievement and liberation. I had been on pills for fourteen years and it was no small accomplishment to not be a pill-popper any more. When my Tourette's inevitably revved up again, I experimented with some alternative therapies – dietary supplements, vitamins, food combining, that sort of thing. Again, no improvement. But I was fine with that. I employed a sunny disposition and just danced along with my tics and blew along with my raspberries.

Slowly, my life began to fall into place. OK, I didn't manage to remain drug free in the end, but just because I found that I had to go back on Efexor in the hope of finding mild relief, it didn't mean that I failed in embracing myself as a Tourettist. Acceptance isn't about giving up. I'll try any safe drug that comes my way in the hope of eradicating some of my exhausting tics. Who wouldn't?

So where does that leave me now? Well, no, I'm not just sitting here madly Touretting myself into a coma, or having such wild obsessive thoughts and desires that I dare not go out for fear of having to carry them out. Nor am I wrapped up in my own misery, or reflecting on what a bad deal life has given me. Those days have gone forever, thankfully.

One huge positive in my life now is that I have my relationship back. It took a long time, lots of space and silence, then lots of talking, but I finally had a reconciliation, a proper one, with Carlo. We're back together again now, and, in a sense, understanding our rift has made our relationship stronger than it ever was; the fact that we overcame the obstacle has, in an uncanny way, left us both feeling more secure. So I'm now conducting a long-distance relationship, popping back to Portugal when I can, and at other times meeting Carlo in London. We're back to enjoying the things about each other that attracted us in the first place. We're loving each other a little more with each passing day and are both certain, beyond any doubt, that this is the love that will never end. Somehow we both know that, and it's a wonderful feeling. Something else I know is that I will never again let my Tourette's stand in the way of something that is so important to me, and the reason for that is because I am no longer at war with myself. I know *exactly* what I am and, even though it took me thirty years to get here, I do truly accept myself. I finally like me.

I try and discipline my days. I do some piano practice, I listen to music, I read, I go out with friends and I laugh and cry as I always did. Having Tourette's has never been a sentence that renders me unable to have fun, and, as I've only now come to appreciate, it's the fun and the joy of life, the laughter, that has probably got me through. I spend a lot of time with Alan and we reminisce, gossip, speculate, play our ever-bungling piano duets and help each other through the multiple humps of life that we know we have to slither over. I even give myself naughty and wicked little Touretty treats too. I do hate supermarkets, but remember the girl who works in my local supermarket, the one whose eye I am desperate to spit in? Well, I force myself to brave all the shelves, products, aisles and stacks every few days or so. I go into that supermarket and check that the girl is working, and am in seventh heaven as I dash around, buying nothing in particular, but relishing the thought of looking temptation quite literally right in the eye and being served by her. It's my way of letting my Tourette's know that it hasn't broken me. And never will.

I don't know what lies in my future, or what it holds, but I'm not worried anymore. I know who I am, so the prospect of starting off again from scratch doesn't faze me in the least. Who knows, I might even try and give a concert one of these days, if I'm feeling brave enough. I'm quite certain I'll dabble with more writing. I've loved penning this memoir, and now ideas for fiction novels are catapulting (obsessively) through my brain, so I feel lucky. I seem to have discovered yet another passion.

But of one thing I'm absolutely sure, and that's the certainty that no matter where I am, whatever I'm doing or how I'm doing it, my Tourette's will always be with me. And that's no longer a daunting prospect for me. I'm a Tourettist and I've lived a colourful life. Did the Tourette's provoke the vibrant shades of dark and light and everything in-between that I've experienced? I just don't know, but I think it must have. Tourette's certainly moulded my personality, it made me the person I am, and despite my wild and wacky compulsions, the physical pain of ticcing all day long and the stubbornness of my busy, busy body, I suppose that, in truth, I'm a happy Tourettist. And it's really time for me to start celebrating that. I'm *not* half a person courtesy of Tourette's syndrome. In fact, I think I'm larger than life, and that suits me just fine.

I was talking to my mother recently about TS and all that goes with it, and she said that if she'd known that in having me, if in giving me Tourette's, she would have ruined my life, then she would never have had children at all.

'But I love life,' I said. 'I love my life.'

And so I do.

So here I sit in London, in my parents' house, in my room with my piano, surrounded by all my music books and recordings, yelping, snorting, grunting, tooth-grinding, nail-biting, buttock-clenching, hyperventilating, blinking, squinting, grimacing, pouting, counting, spitting, touching, knee-bending, calf-flexing, stomach-contracting, laughing and obsessing, dealing with the bombardment of sounds, sights, smells, colours, surfaces to touch, voices and faces that mercilessly rain on me from the real world and experiencing frustration, suppression, anguish, pain, insult, aching, side-splitting-hysteria, nervousness and ultimately a desperate, yet smotheringly chaotic, sense of isolation.

And I feel fine.

Sometimes it seems like I haven't lived at all when I try and look back over my life. It seems that all my hopes, all my passions and all my dreams, have wafted into such a far-off place that I'll never be able to find them again, because I can't really remember what they were. It seems like I left them all behind a thousand years ago. I've come full circle, you see. I'm back to square one.

The future is a blank canvas for me now, but, you know what, I'm ready to paint it.

EPILOGUE

It was when I was lying in bed fighting insomnia one night that I became obsessed with penning my story. I sat up and said to myself, 'Welcome to my world,' and thought about how I might go about explaining life with Tourette's to someone who had no idea about it, how I could try to dispel the myths about the swearing thing, how I could expose the sides of it that people never really get to hear of, how I might try to show that no matter what a Tourettist does, no matter where he or she goes, or how he or she does things, the syndrome is there all the time, an unwelcome guest, but a constant companion.

I became absolutely consumed with memories of the thousands upon thousands of times I've had to stifle my tics, suppress vocal noises, resist my compulsions to touch people and things, absolutely deny myself the opportunity of doing or carrying out a particularly peculiar Tourettism. I kind of relived all the times I've had to excuse myself from a situation and run off to find a private place, just so I could let rip with a wacky Touretty thing that, although bizarre by any normal standards, although monumentally crackpot in itself, gave me a fleeting moment of inner peace, release and satisfaction. I mused over all the excuses I've had to give to justify my often undoubtedly off-the-wall behaviour, excuses given to try to deflect attention away from that which I now wholeheartedly acknowledge is the fundamental me. I recalled reactions from other people when I did tell them that I had TS: some unkind, some sympathetic, but mostly just a blank stare and the assumption that I was simply giving my oddness – madness even – a flowery and affected name. My whole life seems to have been spent explaining, denying, convincing, deflecting, avoiding, agonising and stifling, all with one goal, one single intention: that of somehow being able to portray myself as normal.

I'm not on a mission to show the world how valid Tourettists are as people, or to make everyone aware of Tourette's in order for them to empathise, understand and tread gently around Tourettists, and, by doing so, make them feel even more abnormal than they actually feel. I haven't written this to paint all Tourettists as 'normal' either, for normal is the one thing that they will never be, no matter how hard they try. What I did want, though, was to show how it really *is* to have Tourette's and live with it every single day. And if, at times, my account veered away from the blatant violence of TS, and focused on the more commonplace circumstances of my life, then I am happy, because in doing that, maybe I showed that a life *with* Tourette's doesn't necessarily have to be a life *of* Tourette's. Not all of the time, anyway.

One thing that began to consume me as I was writing this is what impression I was giving of myself. I don't mean whether you thought I was a good or bad guy, or if I was the sort of person you might be able to get along with, but more if you were forming a mental picture of this guy, of me, of the person with Tourette's, and, if you were, what it was. The idea of someone with a shocking neurological condition instantly shoots an image to *my* mind, one of a somehow 'defective' individual, possibly with long greasy hair, a pasty, ghost-like complexion, colossal tortoiseshell spectacles, sitting all wrapped up and hunched, wearing a musty, old green duffel coat and rocking backwards and forwards endlessly. If you then add the Touretty things to that picture, he would be sitting there tooting, barking, gyrating, grimacing, flexing and shaking, jigging away to his own little tune, one that no one else can hear or imagine – a sad little specimen with no place on the plateau of normality.

Every little turn of phrase that I employed to describe my Tourette's took me one step closer to thinking that your picture of me might be something like the description I gave above, and I started to worry. I became concerned that if I told you how my Tourette's really, *really* was, then I would steer you further and further away from seeing that beneath the movements and noises lay all the ingredients for normality. I've led a normal life, one like many millions of other people, probably. One with love, anguish, hopes, disappointments and laughter. The only thing different about me is that I did it all with an enigma of a companion, one that makes me behave very strangely.

I often ask myself if, considering all the torment Tourette's has caused me, I would take a miracle pill to make it all go away should one be offered to me. I'd certainly take a pill that gave me relief, but one to make it vanish entirely? I just don't know. Yes, it's sometimes appalling living with Tourette's, and, yes, it has almost certainly ruined aspects of my life, my prospects and my hopes, things that might have all gone swimmingly if I was Tourette-free. But, having come this far with it beside me, constantly part of me, well, I really don't know how I'd be if it suddenly went away. I don't know if I'd be the same person, whether I'd laugh, whether I'd cry, whether I'd *feel* life in the same way.

I know beyond all doubt that Tourette's has let me see life, experience it, perhaps get a unique slant on things, in a way that many people probably never get near. That's not to put me above anyone else, or to paint myself as though in some wonderfully privileged position. I just experience things rather differently, startlingly so, at times, that's all. Oh it's very easy for you to look at a Tourettist and see the obvious and often entertaining 'isms' of the syndrome, but remember, I, as a Tourettist, am looking out at you, looking out at *your* world, the one that doesn't have tics and noises, and grimaces, and jerking and gyrating, and I have to tell you that *it*, your world, looks very odd to me indeed. I don't just see people going about their business, I see noses coming at me, elbows, eyes, knees, hair, things, things and more things. Things to grab, touch, obsess about touching, things to count, things that zoom lightning fast into my vision, masses of humanity busying themselves in other things and not themselves. I see people who are so at ease with their own bodies and bodily movements that they don't know what it's like to be consciously in touch with every muscle and every bone and every joint of their bodies all of the time. I sometimes see people relaxing in a way that's next to impossible for me, and where they might look at jumpy, fidgety, ticcy me and say, 'Why the hell can't he just relax?', I look at them and think, 'How on earth *can* they relax.' To me, your world is weirder than mine.

It's strange, because I never really feel entirely part of your world, and, in a sense, that makes me feel as though I'm a consummate traveller, floating and breezing through, observing the wonderful and often amusing way you all function, without ever really planting my feet firmly down alongside you and feeling part of things. It's a bit like living in limbo, I suppose, and at least that aspect of having Tourette's isn't in the least bit unpleasant. You see, I don't want to have to deal with the realities of your world, of normal life, because I'm too consumed in dealing with the reality of mine.

If you do ever happen upon a Tourettist on your travels, instead of thinking how weird they happen to be or how out of place they look according to the rules of normality that you live by, perhaps you'll remember that they are probably looking back at you and thinking how very strange you seem, how absolutely alien *you* are.

It's amusing that whatever I'm doing, whether I'm professionally active, exhausted, brimming with joy or shattered by living, people who know me always say the same thing to me at some point.

'Keeping busy?' they ask. 'You've got to keep busy.'

'Oh yes,' I reply. '*Very* busy.'

About the Author

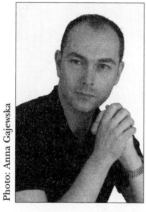

Photo: Anna Gajewska

Nick van Bloss is thirty-eight years old and lives in North London.

His first tic emerged at age seven and he was finally diagnosed with Tourette's syndrome at twenty-one. Trained as a pianist at London's Royal College of Music, he has won numerous competitions, played concerts, taught, examined and given master-classes in the UK and internationally.

Now 'retired' as a musician, he considers himself a professional Tourettist. *Busy Body* is his first book.